A Tale of Two Teachers

How Ralph Millard and Paul Tessier changed the face of Plastic Surgery

by S. Anthony Wolfe, M.D. and Erin M. Wolfe, M.D.

DORRANCE
PUBLISHING CO
EST. 1920
PITTSBURGH, PENNSYLVANIA 15238

Dorrance Publishing Co
585 Alpha Drive
Pittsburgh, PA 15238
Visit our website at *www.dorrancebookstore.com*

ISBN: 979-8-88729-430-8
eISBN: 979-8-88729-930-3

Prologue

This monograph is a hybrid: it is both biographical and autobiographical, documenting the influence that two remarkable plastic surgeons have had on the specialty of plastic surgery, changing it forever with their revolutionary ingenuity and audacity. It is partially a surgical text, partially a documentary of two men's lives.

One can chart a direct line from the first generation of plastic surgeons, Morestin and Gillies, through Millard and Tessier, the second generation, through the third generation of myself and my colleagues, ending with the 4th generation of my daughter, Erin, who is just beginning her plastic surgery residency. Each generation has learned from the prior, broadening and deepening the scope of the specialty.

From Millard, we will show how our dissatisfaction with one-stage bilateral cleft repairs led us to the adoption of staged rotation advancements, "bilateral Millards," with better nasal and lip results, and also better maxillary growth, and the importance of the skeletal platform correction before secondary correction of the lip and nose in cleft patients, the cocaine nose, dealing with lining deficiency in nasal reconstruction, face lifting, breast reconstruction and tube pedicles, which may not be completely extinct.

From Tessier, we will show some of his unmatched results, and show the use of distraction osteogenesis in secondary maxillary advancement, a procedure that came into use after Tessier's retirement. We will show our use of his approach for the treatment of enophthalmos and exophthalmos, and our treatment of vertical orbital dystopias, now with a minimally invasive approach, a logical extension of Tessier's approach, the treatment of hypotelorism, another logical extension, the "mask lift," oracular clefts. As well as the importance of primary bone grafting in pan facial fractures. Also from Tessier, orthomorphic surgery, the "Tools and Techniques," the James Barret Brown award-winning PRS Supplement on bone grafts.

On the biographical side, there will be an examination of the similarities of the two innovators who were disruptive, and revolutionary, and initially unaccepted in their own countries, but then accepted, respected as world leaders, and recipients of every available honor.

And their differences - Millard was a prolific author of books and journal publications. Tessier, because he was so self-critical, wrote very little. His early work, for instance on the treatment of enophthalmos, was in French, and therefore unknown and unappreciated by the English-speaking audience.

Tessier wrote an entire book on the anatomy of the major craniofacial malformations, with patient photographs, drawings, and x-rays. When 3-dimensional scans became available he insisted that each malformation have one. The book was never published.

A Tale of Two Teachers

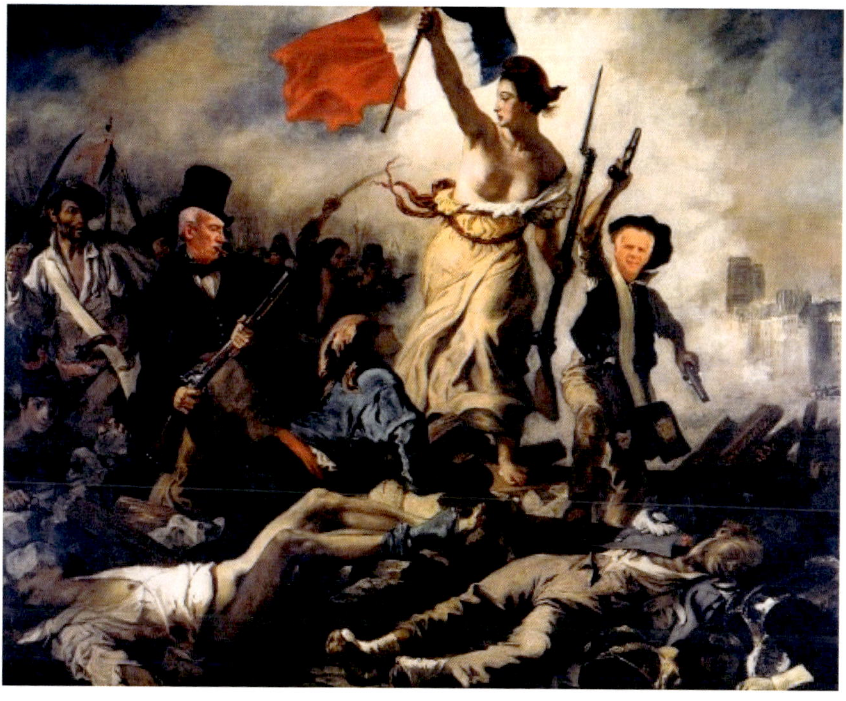

How Ralph Millard and Paul Tessier changed the face of Plastic Surgery

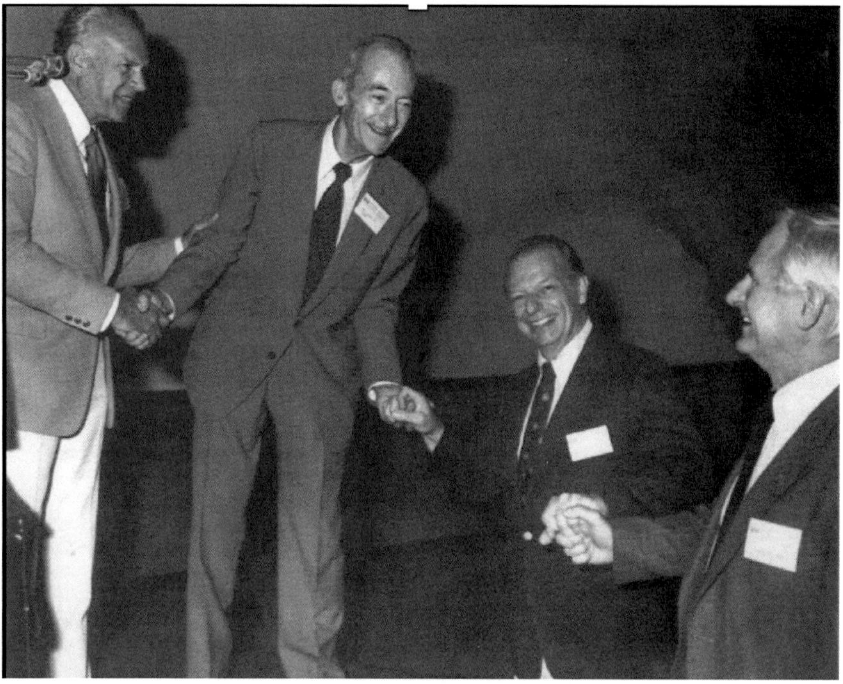

Ralph Millard and Paul Tessier together as Keynote Speakers at the International Society of Plastic Surgery meeting in Montreal in 1983; the others are Bob Chase and Bernie O'Brien.

D. Ralph Millard, Jr.,M.D. 1919-2011
Aet. 92

When I was an HMS-3 (third year student at the Harvard Medical School), I was considering what I would like to do in medicine. Surgery was a natural choice, my grandfather and uncle were both urologists, but sadly for my grandfather, I was not interested in urology. Maybe neurosurgery.

I had had a rotation on the Neurosurgical Service at the Massachusetts General Hospital. On rounds it seemed that most of the patients were and remained comatose. And I saw a chief resident pour hydrogen peroxide into a brain abscess, which had a vigorous reaction of brain and abscess bubbling, certainly the end of the line for that young woman. Neurosurgery was not for me.

I wanted something that required dexterity and craftsmanship. I stayed in the general surgery program at the Peter Bent Brigham Hospital in Boston, headed by the Moseley Professor at Harvard, the legendary Frannie Moore, who was a surgical superstar not because of his surgical skills, but since he had been on the cover of Time Magazine for his work on the metabolic care of surgical patients. General Surgery was fun but somehow limited.

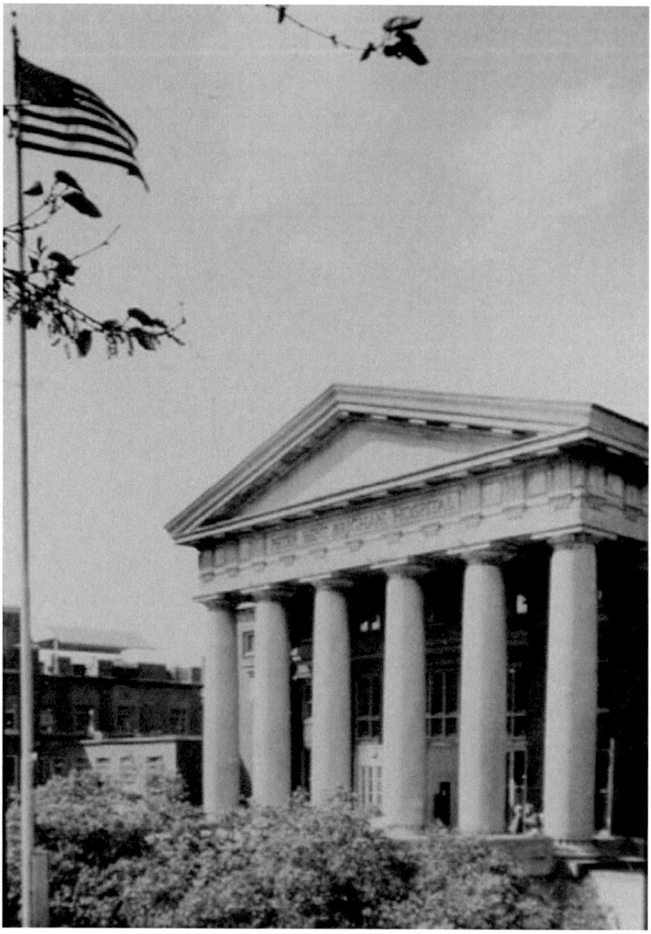

The Peter Bent Brigham Hospital, now Brigham and Women's.

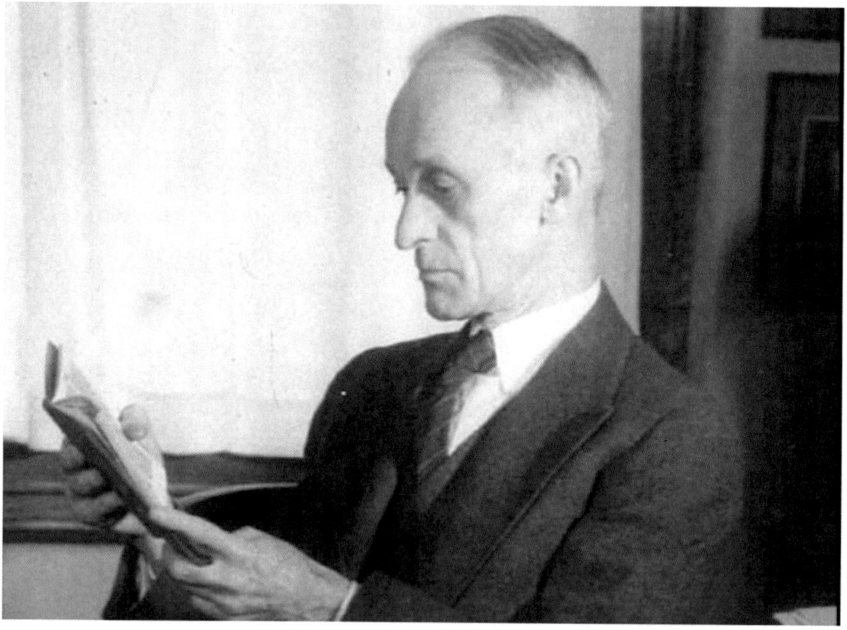

Harvey Cushing, the father of Neurosurgery and the first Surgeon-in-Chief of the Brigham, at his desk.

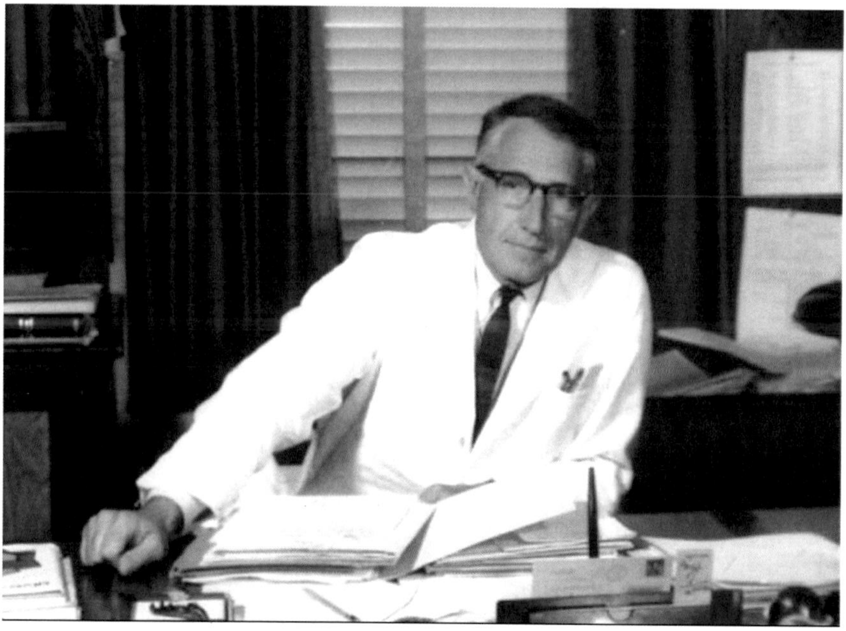

Dr. Moore, sitting at the same desk.

Bob Goldwyn came over once from the Beth Israel and did an abdominoplasty, but that was it.

Joe Murray did some major head and neck cancer surgery, but with hardly any reconstruction.

I was left to acquaint myself with plastic surgery by looking through The Journal of Plastic and Reconstructive Surgery. One author stood out for his publications on cleft lip and nasal surgery: D Ralph Millard, Jr.

Millard's training

Millard's training came at a difficult time to be a trainee. His medical school class at Harvard in 1944 was condensed to 3 years during WWII Following graduation he spent 9 months in a pediatric surgery program at Boston Children's Hospital, and then went into the Navy and thence to Vanderbilt where he entered a general surgery residency.

During his time at Vanderbilt in 1947, Sir Harold Gillies, in Tennessee for The American Association of Plastic Surgeons meeting, paid a visit to Beverly Douglas, the Head of Plastic surgery at Vanderbilt. The young Millard was very impressed and asked Gillies if he could come to Gillies unit. Gillies, after a brief conversation said yes, but added that he was on the verge of retirement, and suggested Millard contact Rainsford Mowlem instead.

At that time, it was customary for a renowned surgeon to charge a visitor to his service, Millard wrote Gillies asking if the $500 from his GI Bill would suffice, but received no answer.

He then simply showed up and was accepted and spent a year assisting Gillies. When he had free time he visited other surgeons such as Pomfret Kilner and Archibald McIndoe, and he had tea with Victor Veau in Paris several months before his death.

Millard then returned to the US, where he had managed to find a slot in the residency program at Washington University in St. Louis under James Barret Brown, who had been the head of all plastic surgery for the US Military during WW11. Apparently, Millard heckled Brown once too often with questions, particularly ones including what Gillies would have done. Brown fired him after 6 months of this.

Millard then found a position as the first resident of the new program at Baylor in Houston, and this, along with 6 months with Claire Straith in Detroit (a rhinoplasty surgeon) provided enough training to satisfy The American Board of Plastic Surgery

Following this, in 1955 Millard was drafted again and sent to Korea, where in a lull in the fighting he ran a busy service reconstructing Koreans with facial injuries, one evening waking up from a snooze, he had the idea for the rotation-advancement lip repair. He said the procedure came to him in his half sleep.

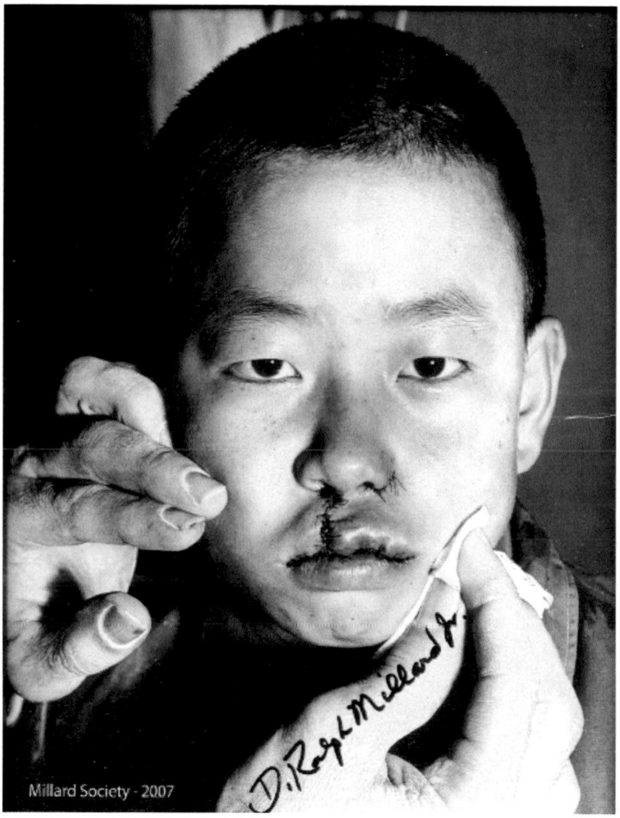

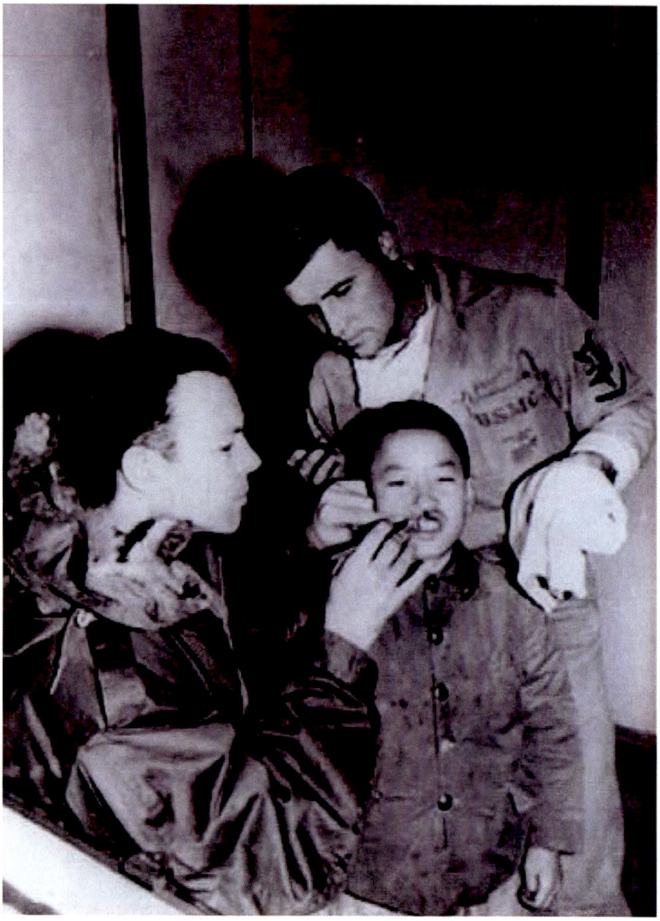

Millard's first rotation advancement performed in Korea.

Following this spell in Korea, he returned to Gillies and did the lion's share of the work on their book, Gillies and Millard, *The Principles and Art of Plastic Surgery*. This was an unconventional medical textbook, containing wit and humor, and many complex reconstructions. It still remains the best source of information about forehead flaps, and contains the first published account of an osseous genioplasty.

Brad Cannon of the Mass General was asked by Little Brown to review the book, and he responded that it should never be published, and that there was no place for humor in a medical textbook.

A Radical Rotation in Single Harelip

D. Ralph Millard, Jr., m.d., *Miami, Florida*

Millard published the rotation advancement in a general surgical journal, not a plastic one.

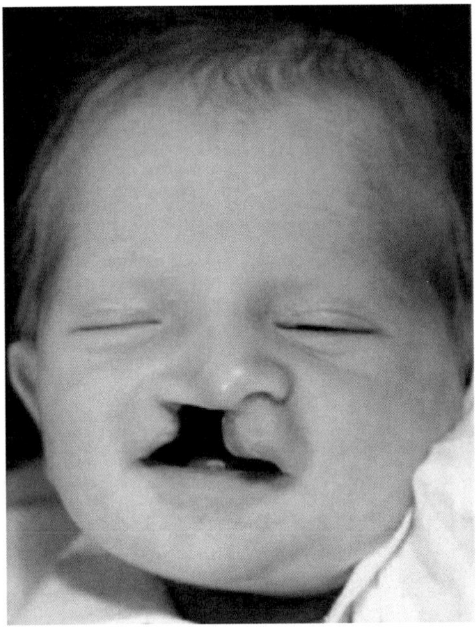

Here is a wide unilateral cleft with Millard's markings for a rotation advancement.

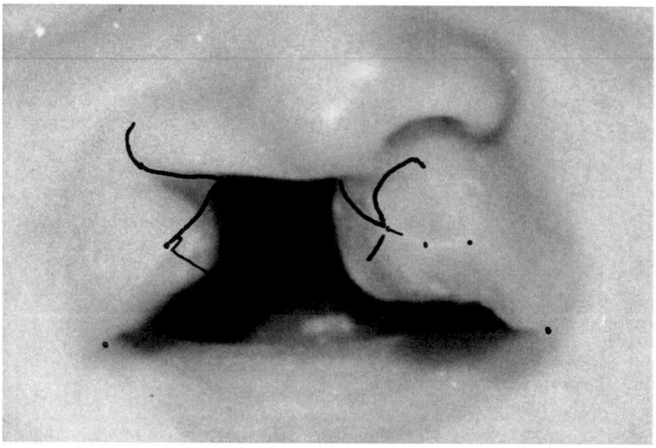

Millard carries the incision further around the ala than I find necessary, I have never used the little white roll flap and Millard abandoned it.

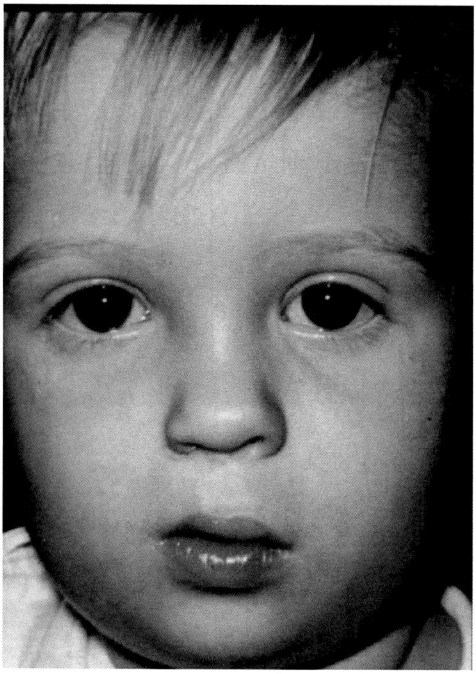

Millard's result: the lip is shorter on the cleft side, but the Cupid's bow is preserved, and the lip scar is in the position of the normal philtra column. Critics say that it is "cut as you go" which is true. There are no triangles or numbers to guide you.

There follow a number of my unilaterals, taken out of the Time narrative. I have deviated from Millard's depiction slightly by not going as far around with the alar base incision. Also, the nasal correction was the McComb closed method rather than Millard's direct open approach with a vestibular incision. And, I had available NAM—nasoalveolar moulding, which made everything easier and permitted an alveolar closure.

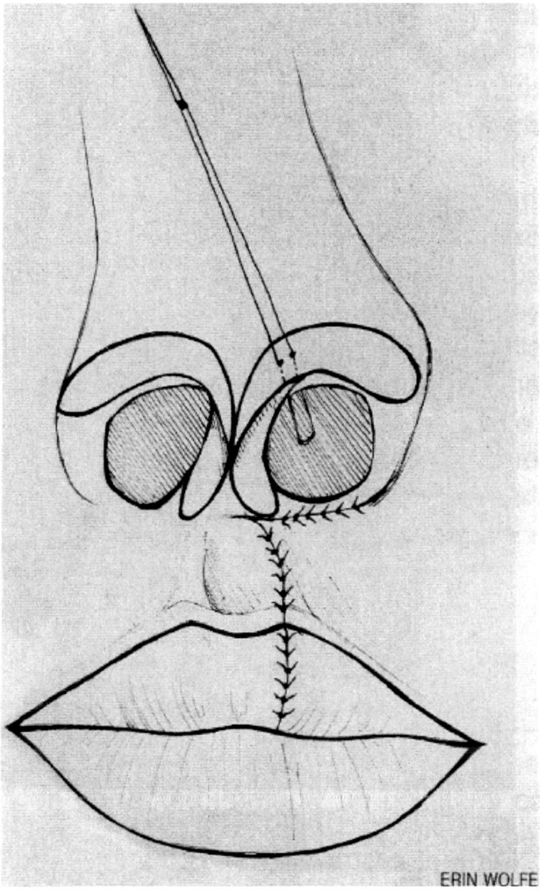

McComb suture elevating left alar cartilage.

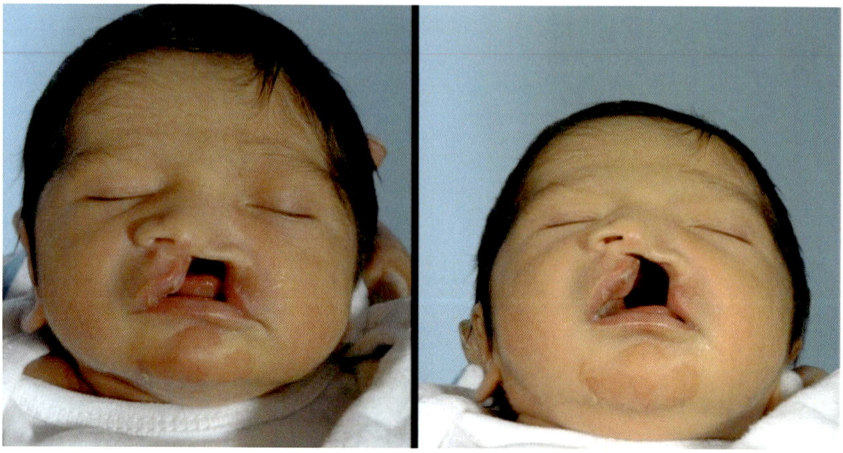

Complete cleft with wide alveolar gap and alar slump before 5 months of treatment with NAM (naso-alveolar moulding).

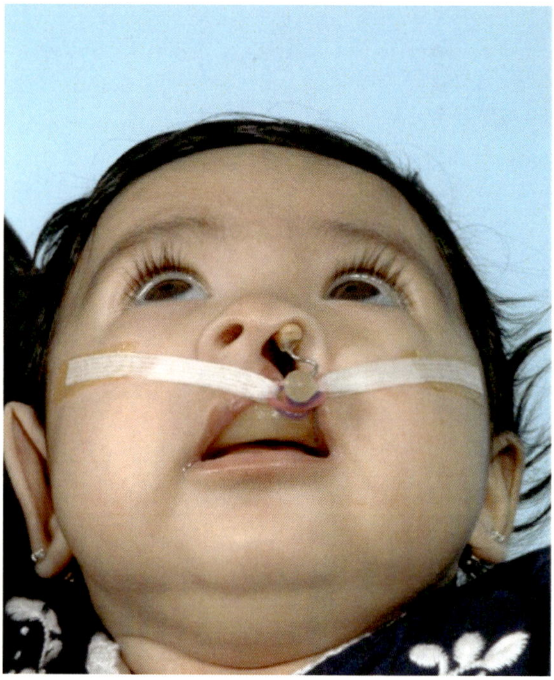

NAM in progress.

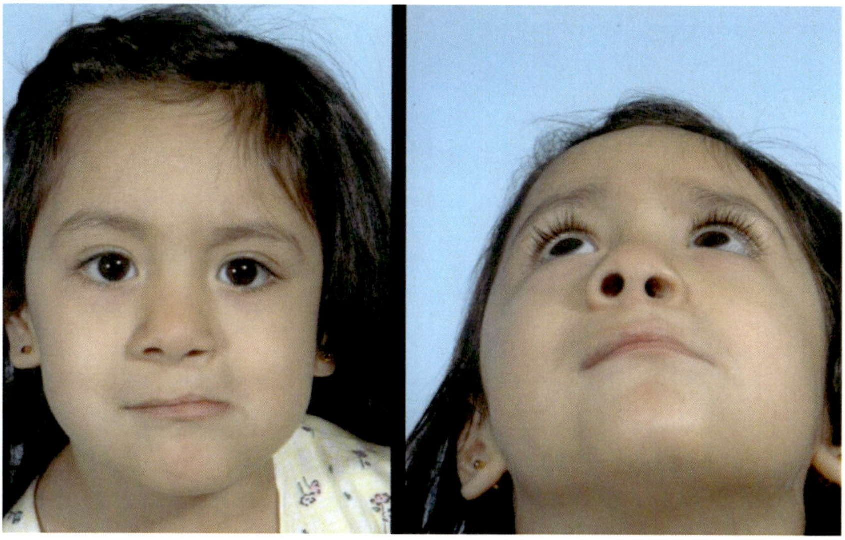

Result at age 4. Good nasal correction but small vestibular web in cleft side nares. Lip is slightly underrotated which makes it short on the cleft side. Millard taught his trainees to be critical even of a good result.

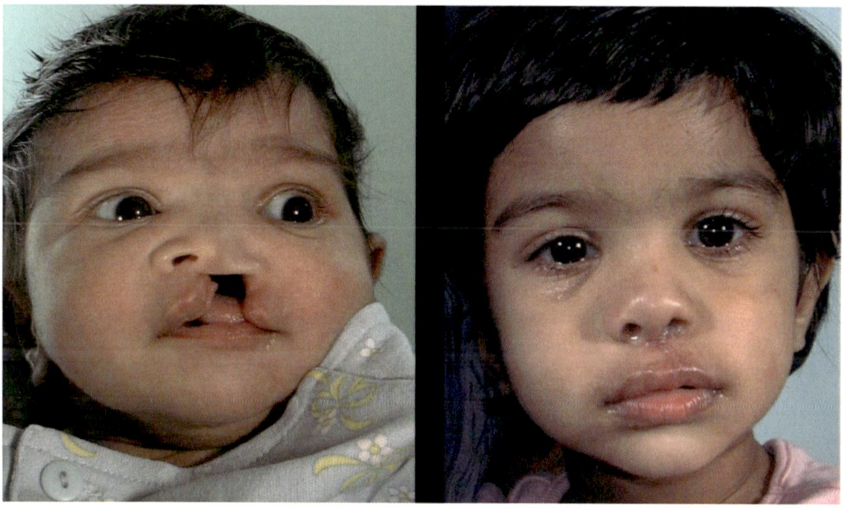

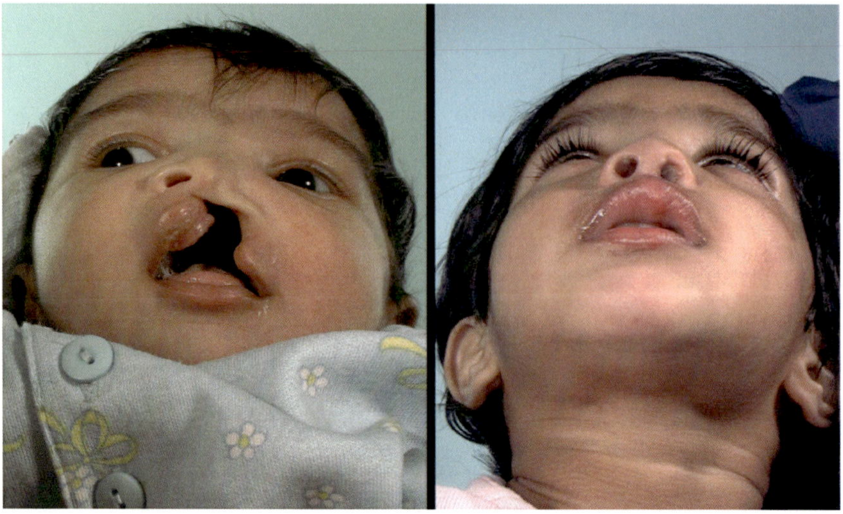

Better result but small vestibular web still seen.

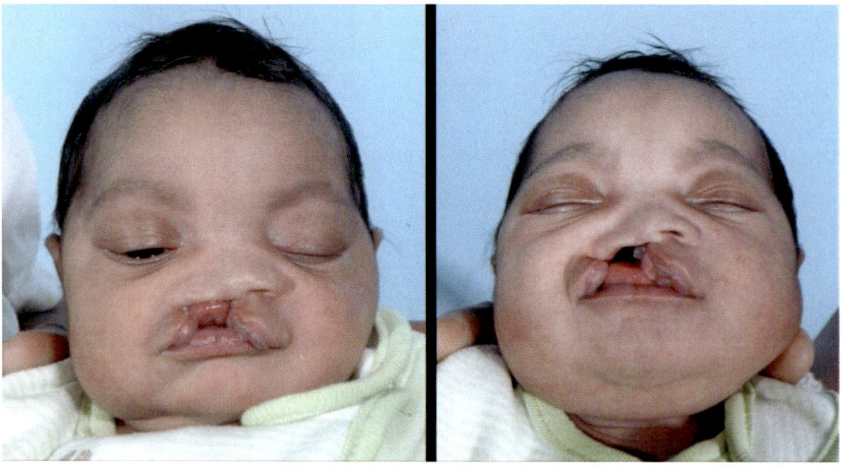

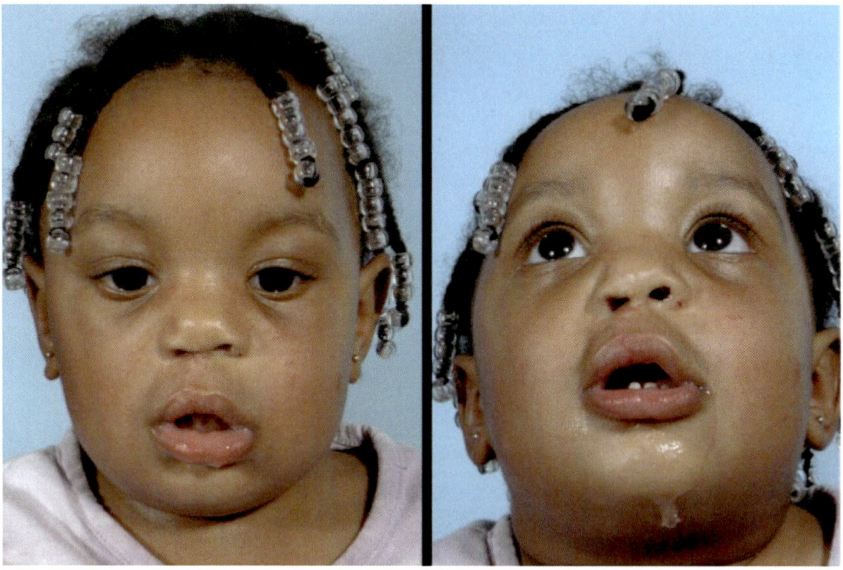

Very wide cleft with major alar slump. Good result with the white roll.

Millard essentially put together his own training program by piecing together residency spots where he could find them. He was disruptive and impertinent when faced with a self-satisfied teacher, and he bucked the system. It is no surprise that his stay was short in some programs.

His treatment of his own residents probably reflected the treatment he had received from Gillies. Call it tough love.

Having decided to pursue plastic surgery, I asked Joe Murray for his opinion on which programs to apply to. He mentioned NYU with John Converse and Johns Hopkins under Milton Edgerton. I asked about Millard and got somewhat of a negative assessment—his results were so good that he was not to be trusted and he was somewhat of a showoff. I didn't ask Dr. Murray about the plastic surgery residency program that he was planning on opening at Brigham/Children's.

The Brigham at that time had a Travelling Fellowship for senior residents, which had a stipend and two weeks of time to visit any program they wished. I took that as an opportunity to go to interview for plastic surgery residencies, I wrote to NYU, Hopkins, and Miami.

Miami was not listed in the Green Book listing residencies, but nevertheless I wrote to Dr. Millard to see if there was a residency in Miami. I received an invitation to come for an interview from Dr. Converse and Edgerton, taking an afternoon, and a letter from a Dr. John Devine for an interview in Miami which would take three days.

I recall the interview with Dr Converse. He had on a tailored suit and sat behind his desk in a somewhat dimly lit office. I can't recall much about the interview, but he said I could find out about the program from the residents—of whom there were 9. I had the sense that there was a large staff of residents with not many patients to care for.

Next was Hopkins. Here the interview included going to a teaching session, having an interview with a member of the staff who did hand surgery, and then meeting Dr. Edgerton for lunch in the staff dining room.

After lunch we walked across a courtyard, and he told me that a surgeon in France had done some interesting work with facial advancement, and that he was planning to do the procedure on one of his own patients. Remember this for an episode later in the book.

Finally, there was the trip to Miami. One day with Dr. Millard in his office, one day with the residents at their grand rounds, and one day watching Dr. Millard operate.

He did a unilateral cleft lip. I looked over his left shoulder and was impressed with his fluidity and the way he handled tissue. When the case was finished and we were leaving the operating room he asked me, "What did you think of that?" I answered that it was very interesting, and that he didn't throw anything away and had a use for every bit of tissue.

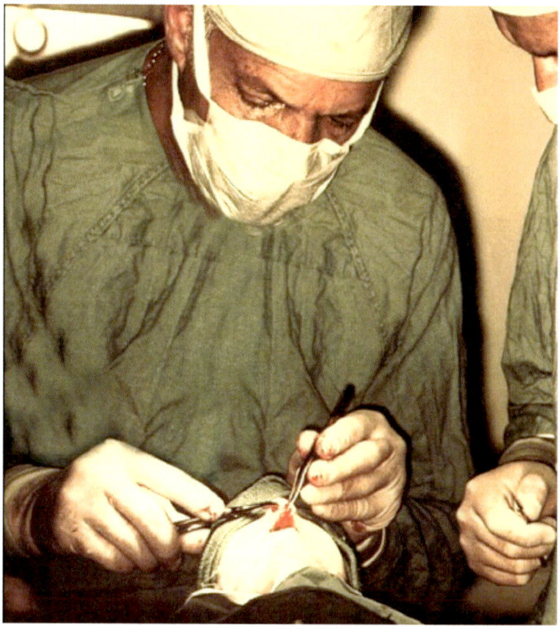

Fig. Millard suturing a cleft with his Gillies needle holder.

Apparently, that was the right answer. We went down to the cafeteria for lunch.

He was ahead of me in the line, and turned partly around and said, somewhat out of the corner of his mouth, there's a job here for you if you want it.

Without hesitation I accepted. Later I received notice from NYU and Hopkins that I had been accepted by those programs, but I had already made my decision: Miami. This was before the match.

Craniofacial surgery. When I was a medical student, our class was taken by bus to the Fernald School, in Waltham, on the outskirts of Boston.

Originally founded as "The Massachusetts School for the Feeble-Minded," it was closely linked to the American eugenics movement, which in turn had links to a more sinister movement in Nazi Germany.

In spite of the original name of the institution, over half of the inmates were of normal intelligence, and were there due to their deformity

We were taken to an auditorium and on the stage were paraded a variety of patients with severe craniofacial anomalies including Apert,

Treacher Collins, Crouzon, Down's syndrome and other facial malformations. None of the patients had been operated on, since at that time (1963) there was little surgery available other than silicone implants.

It was standard practice then to institutionalize patients with severe facial deformities, with the thought that this would spare the parents the difficulty of bringing up a severely deformed child.

After years of scandal, Fernald School was eventually closed for good in 2014.

In my last year at the Brigham, already accepted into a plastic surgery residency, I went to Montreal to the meeting of the American Society of Plastic and Reconstructive Surgery. This was in 1971 and was the first time a French Surgeon named Paul Tessier spoke in North America.

I was floored by his results and knew immediately that this was the type of surgery I wanted to do. I wrote Tessier a letter in French asking if I could come to Paris to learn from him. I got no response to that letter, so I asked Millard if he could write a note to Tessier for me. Tessier had visited Millard in the late 1960's in Miami in one of his visits to prominent surgeons in the US, Mexico, and England. This did the trick, and Millard received a note saying that I would be welcome.

Off to Miami.

While in Boston I met someone who said that they knew of a person in Miami who might have a cottage to rent. Douglas Erickson lived in a DiGarmo house on 7 acres at the junction of Douglas (37th Avenue) and Main Highway out of Coconut Grove. He was frequently out of town (Maine, his yacht, Europe) and wanted someone to stay in his guest house. I wrote him. I flew to Miami and met Mr. Erickson and his wife Irina, who it turned out was of white Russian background. I passed muster and the cottage (tin roof, screened in front porch, one bedroom and a small kitchen was my home for the next two years—for $300 a month). There was a painting of a mermaid riding the waves on the ceiling of the bedroom.

I left my parents' home in Northern Virginia, the old 356 Porsche I had bought for $3000 from someone in Maryland packed to the hilt with my belongings, and drove non-stop except for gas stops to Miami. Close to a thousand miles.

I can't recall where I went first - to the plastic surgery office in Jackson Memorial Hospital, where Evelyn Shields was the secretary who ran the service (and in all aspects) or to Dr. Millard's office at 1444 NW 14th Avenue. This building was only a few blocks away from Jackson, close enough to be considered part of the medical campus. It had a red tile roof, Spanish style, with a small bell tower.

There was a lot adjacent to it for parking. In the foyer there was a painting of what appeared to be an Italian seaside village and then the receptionists window. Pre-op patients would be directed to one waiting room to the left, post-ops to a separate waiting room to the right. In one of the waiting rooms was a full size painting of Gaspar Tagliacozzi.

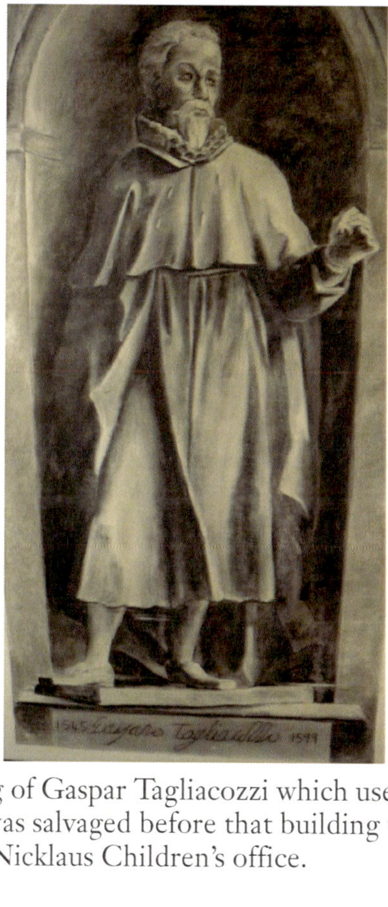

Life-sized painting of Gaspar Tagliacozzi which used to be in the 14th Avenue office. It was salvaged before that building was torn down and now hangs in the Nicklaus Children's office.

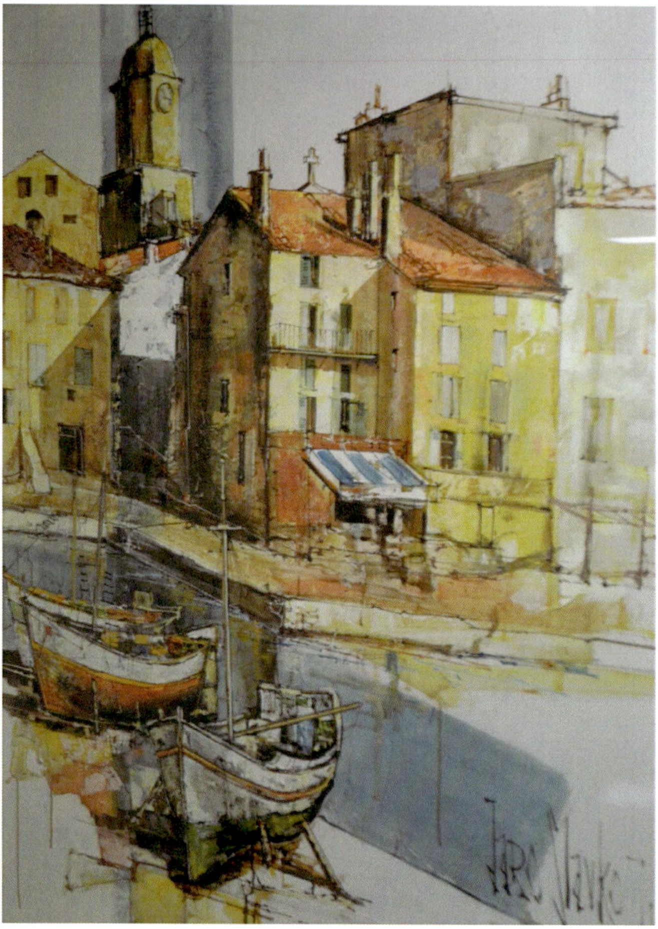

Painting which hung in the foyer of the 14th Avenue office of Italian seaport.

The plastic surgery staff service was located on Woodard 2, which has subsequently been torn down for construction of a new building. When the Lenny Bruce Story was being filmed, with Dustin Hoffman, Woodard was selected because it perfectly resembled a run-downward in a municipal hospital in the 1950's.

There was Evelyn's office, an adjacent meeting room where rounds could be held, 6 or 7 hospital beds, and a small operating room where the residents could do anything that could be done under local. Face-lifts, blepharoplasties rhinoplasties, you name it.

This was the staff service—with a senior resident in charge, and the new junior resident his subordinate. An LPN named Dee Harrison helped with the surgeries.

There were 2 residents a year, one of the other residents was at the VA hospital, and the other on Dr. Millard's private service.

Dr. Millard rarely helped the resident on the staff service, although he liked to get involved with cleft lips and nasal reconstruction. The teaching got done at rounds, where the residents would bring their preop patients, and present a surgical plan, often criticized by Dr. Millard.

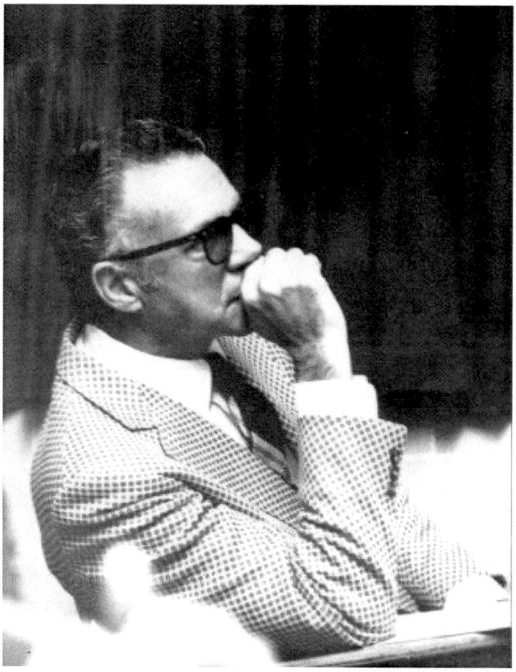

Dr. Millard, inscrutably behind his dark glasses at rounds.

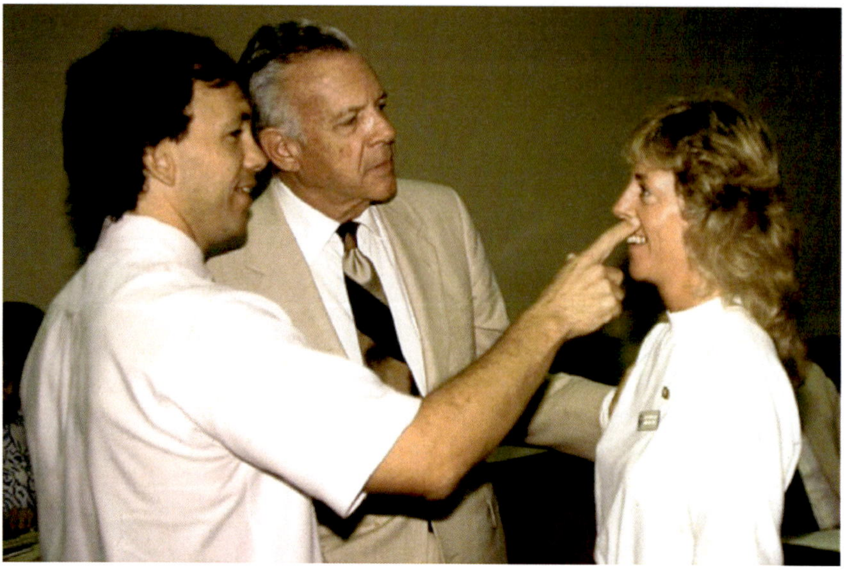

Dr. Millard examining a patient with resident (Leo McCafferty).

At the end of training, residents were expected to put together presentation of the cases they had done. *One notable resident, Geoff Buncke, came to his presentation bringing two slide projectors, with the advance buttons attached to a pair of sandals, a black case was opened and there was saxophone. Geoff didn't say a word but started playing the theme from The Pink Panther, with the slides behind advanced by his toes, saying breast reconstruction, facial fracture, etc. Dr. Millard was taken aback for sure but being a practical joker himself didn't say a word.*

Aside from Dr Millard's advice at rounds, the residents were pretty much on their own. The only other person who could be considered faculty was Steve Cooley, who did hand surgery and had been trained by Littler. Steve was a severe introvert and might do a 3-hour case and not say a word. He would leave Miami for several months a t a time as crew on a racing yacht. He later committed suicide.

John Devine handled all of the minutiae, paperwork and correspondence that Millard didn't want to deal with. John had been a general surgeon in Roanoke, Virginia, and at age 65 decided that he wanted to be a plastic surgeon. He managed to have Millard grant him an interview, in which Millard told John that taking a residency at 65 was a pipe dream, and to forget it. John was persistent and when Millard had an opening for a fellow, he took John.

John worked his tail off as fellow, and at age 66 Millard took him as the oldest resident on record, a distinction that I am sure still stands.

Plastic surgery covered the emergency room and there was a good bit of facial trauma to care for. We had only wire for osteosyntheses, and the Georgiade head frame for midface fractures.

On New Year's Eve of 1971, when I was the senior resident, I got paged to come to the OR. When I arrived, I saw a man struggling to sit up, while an anesthesia resident was trying get him supine to intubate him. I said stop. He continued. The man had an airway when sitting, but was drowning in blood and secretions when supine.

(This was how so many soldiers died in WWII, when they were sitting or lying face down, they had an airway, but when a corpsman put them in the supine position the patient lost his airway and died.)

I moved the protesting anesthesiologist aside and did a tracheostomy under local anesthesia.

This was Richard L_____, a good old boy from north Florida, who had had too much to drink celebrating the New Year and ran his Pontiac GTO into a cement bridge abutment. This was a true craniofacial case, with the face separated from the cranium.

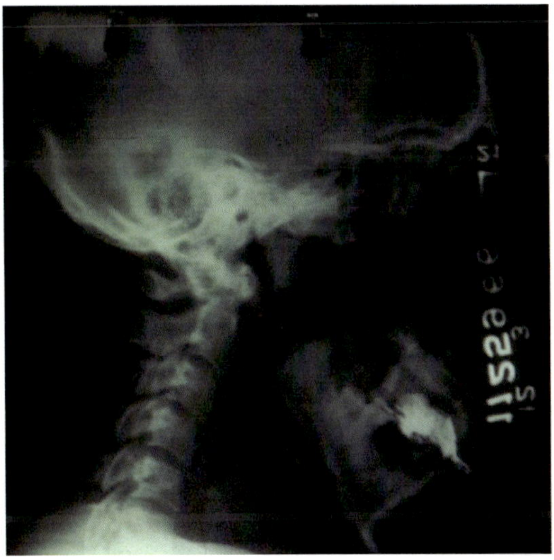

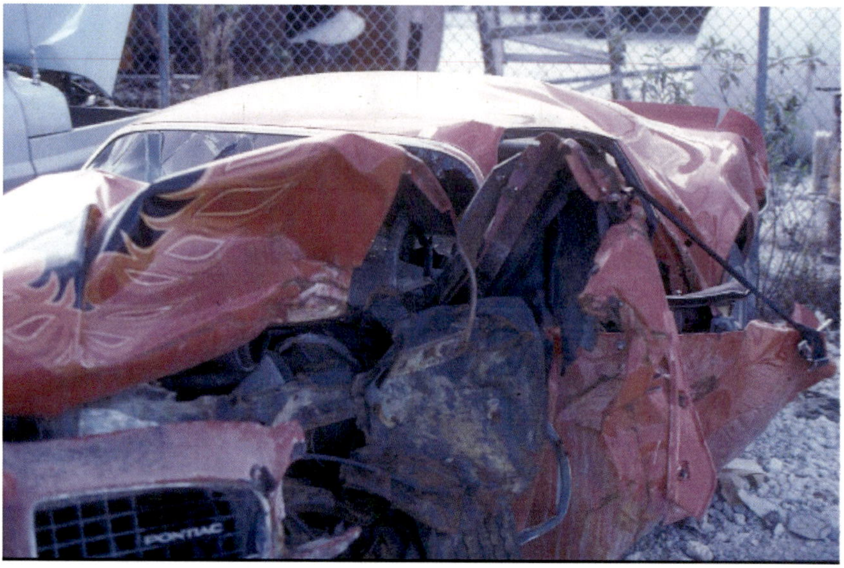
PONTIAC

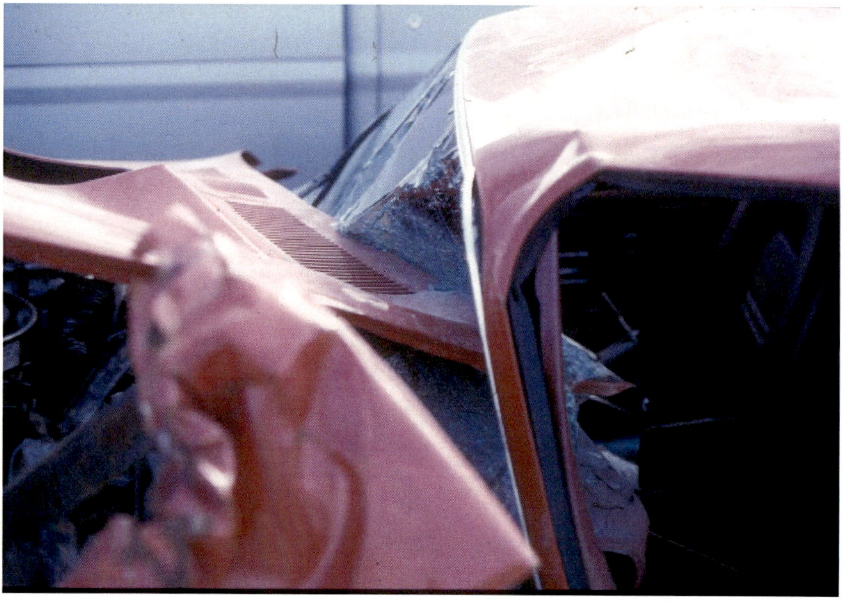

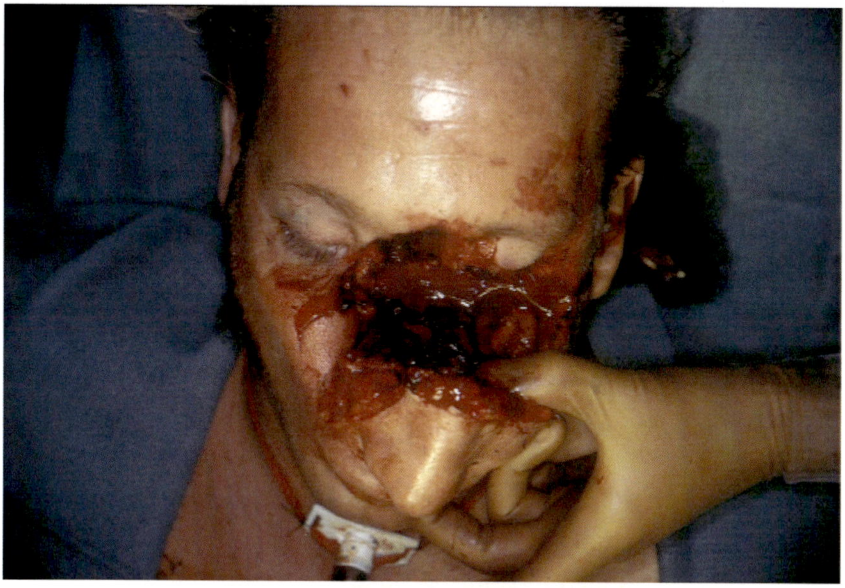

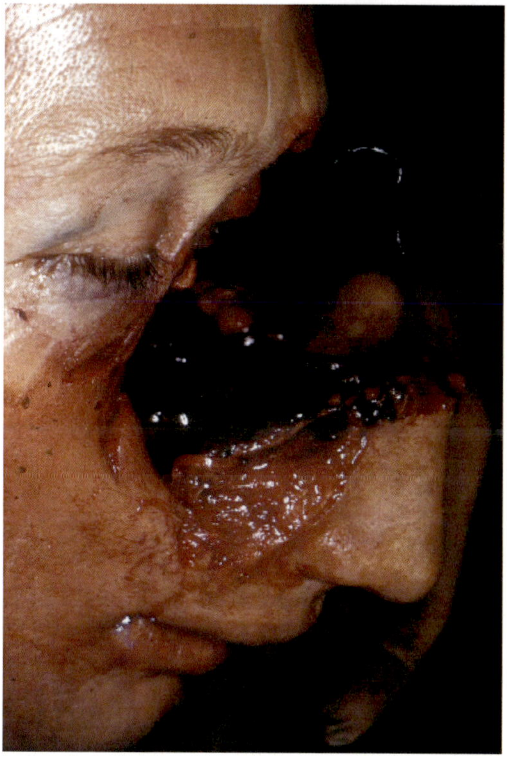

Left globe ruptured, right intact.

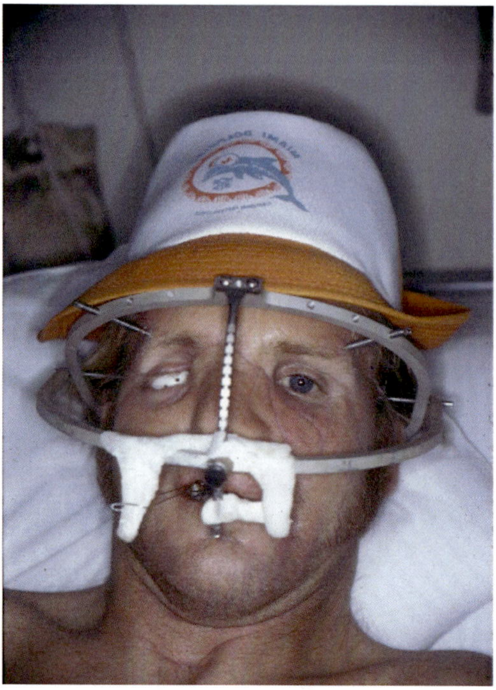

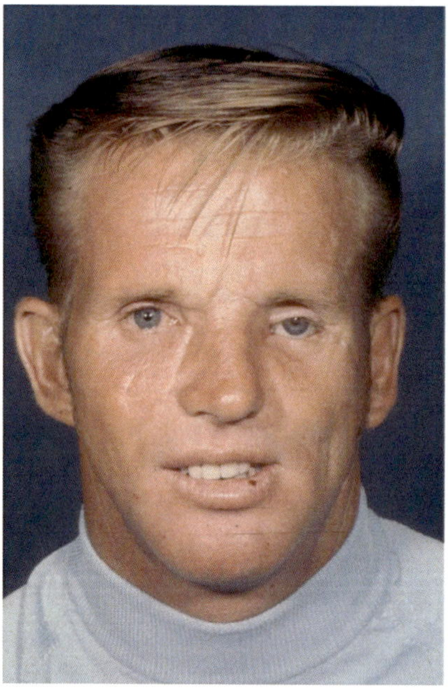

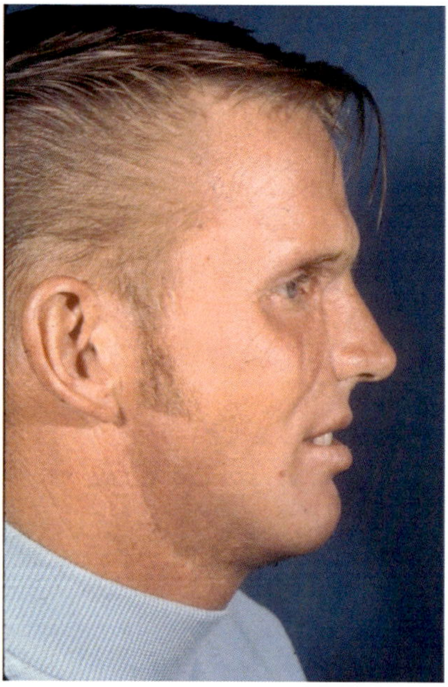

The posterior edge of the hood came through the windshield like a guillotine, inflicting a Le Fort 3 laceration and almost separating his face from his skull.

The treatment he received was standard for that time. The only imaging available was an AP and lateral x-ray of the face and neck.

After the tracheostomy, I wired as many of the fractures as I could identify through small incisions. Arch bars were applied and intermaxillary fixation established. A Georgiade head frame was placed and the maxilla put on traction.

Due to a shift in the maxilla, he ended up with a crossbite. This should have been treated by a Le Fort 1. I asked the head of oral surgery for his opinion, and without any discussion he scheduled him for an extraoral vertical osteotomy—the wrong operation since it moved the mandible off of the facial midline. To the maxilla which had not been properly reduced.

I was proud of the result but viewed with present day standards it is mediocre. The left orbit is dystopic, there is not a proper medial canthopexy and the occlusion is off the facial midline.

Millard did not have much to say about this case, since he was largely a soft tissue doctor. He had published a paper with Walter Garst on primary mandible reconstruction with a forehead flap covering a rib graft after mandibular resection for cancer. This was a pioneering paper, one of the first about primary reconstruction, but this procedure was halted after the general surgeons began using preoperative radiotherapy, and there were a number of infections.

Walter Garst was a Virginian trained in the Jackson General Surgery program where he worked with Dr. Millard on these jaw reconstruction cases and went to Columbia Presbyterian for his first year of plastic surgery. Dr. Millard was just taking over the plastic surgery residency from Gil Snyder, (fresh out of his residency at Hopkins) who was the first Chief of Plastic Surgery. Dean Warren, the Chief of Surgery, hired Millard as "temporary" Chief. Millard retained his "temporary" Chiefship for 25 years. Millard retained his “temporary”

Chiefship for 25 years. He was the only surgeon on staff who was not a full-time employee of the hospital, a fact that caused a good bit of resentment from the others and weakened Millard politically.

Millard fired one of Snyder's residents and kept Peter Stokely as the other. He invited Walter Garst to come to Miami to finish his plastic training, and then took him as an associate. Walter did mostly face lifts, but he helped me do a few radical neck dissections, and forehead flaps.

The first orthognathic cases and the importance of dentistry.

I saw in the clinic a Columbian airline stewardess who had been in a plane crash and fractured her maxilla. She had Class 3 malocclusion, so I referred her to Sam Berkowitz, the orthodontist for the cleft team. He told me that she would need a Le Fort 1 osteotomy and maxillary advancement. I had never seen a Le Fort 1, and one had never been done at Jackson. I read what I could find in the literature—mostly by Hugo Obwegeser of Zurich and went ahead with her operation.

There was a nasal intubation, with Berkowitz's orthodontic brackets with hooks and a rigid arch wire, in place. There was extensive subperiosteal dissection—difficult due to scarring, osteotomy with the Lindemann burr and osteotomes and mobilization with Rowe forceps. I managed to get her maxilla into the occlusal splint that Sam had made and kept her in intermaxillary fixation for 6 weeks with a satisfactory result. This was the first le Fort 1 osteotomy done at Jackson Memorial Hospital, and I went on to do several hundred more with Sam over the years. Seeing Tessier in Paris do many Le Fort 1's made it much easier for me.

I also saw in the clinic a woman who was interested in a breast augmentation. She also had fairly pronounced mandibular prognathism. I asked her if she would like her jaw corrected, and she said "sure, yes, I was interested in getting that corrected, but didn't know it was possible."

Again, to the literature, and again to Obwegeser. One problem was that Jackson did not have the proper instruments. I went to the instrument repair shop and had them alter some old instruments to make channel retractors and other instruments that were needed.

I used a Lindemann side cutting burr with small osteotomes, and fortunately she had a fairly thick mandible that I was able to split without comminution. Wire osteosynthesis. Again, splint by Berkowitz. The patient had a good occlusal and aesthetic result and was not concerned by the numb lip that she had on one side. This was the first sagittal split performed at Jackson.

These were the first two orthognathic cases done at Jackson, by a resident who had never seen either operation before. That would be unheard of today.

First contact with Tessier

Tessier was operating in Chicago in 1973, when I was still a resident. I went up to watch. I can't recall what operation I was, and I doubt if Tessier had any idea who I was.

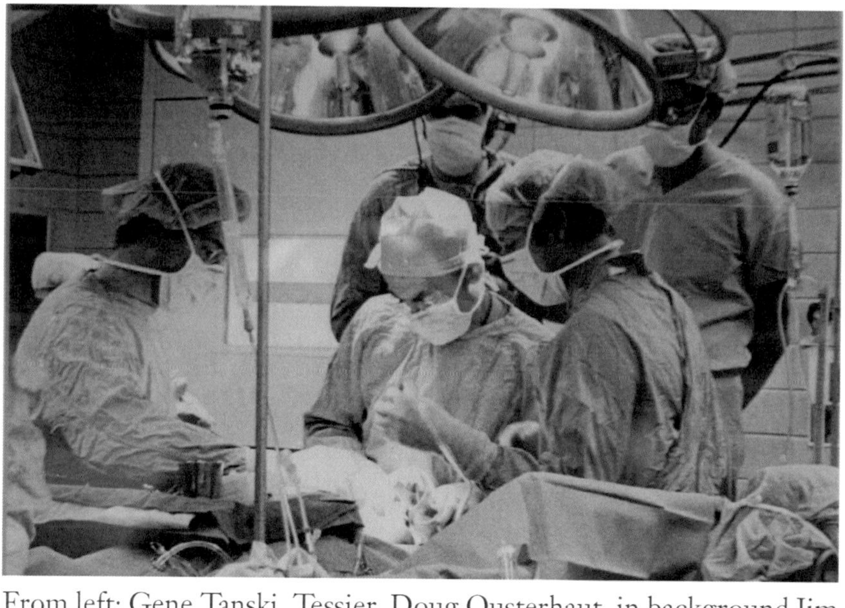

From left: Gene Tanski, Tessier, Doug Ousterhaut, in background Jim Fletcher, ex-Miami photographer, SAW.

A job. By this time, towards the end of my residency I was all set to go to Paris but had no further plans. I was in Millard's office when he came up and asked me if I had any further plans. Nope. He then said that he could use someone to do bones, and I had a job if I was interested.

Sure, I said. Thus began an association which lasted 25 years with no written contract or even handshake. His accountant Anne Cohen would collect for all of the surgery I did and I think I got $70,000 a year at the beginning. When it became evident that I was bringing in much more that the $70,000, we changed the agreement so that I paid a fixed amount for my share of rent and expenses and had a considerable surge in my income.

Henry "Budd" Menn who was a very busy Mohs surgeon who would bring many of his extensive skin cancer patients to our office to discuss preoperatively. Between Millard and I, there was almost a forehead flap weekly.

Two of Millard's trainees, Gary Burget, a resident, and Fred Menick, a fellow, after Millard became the acknowledged new world leaders in nasal reconstruction.

Millard was the pioneer in breast reconstruction, using tube pedicles from abdominoplasty redundancy, before the introduction of the TRAM flap. And he was savaged by the general surgeons who felt that breast reconstruction would mask any possible recurrences. He worked with pediatric surgeons to develop a muscle sphincter for imperforate anus, and with the general surgeons to treat patients with skin grafted eviscerated bowel to dissect the skin grafts from the bowel and close the large abdominal hernia.

Millard was always writing either a paper or a book, and the resident on his service did a good bit of the footwork and ended up being a coauthor. Millard wrote everything on yellow legal pads, sitting on the balcony of his bedroom in Baypoint, and each morning would bring in a few more pages for the secretary to transcribe. I helped him a good bit with his 3-volume oeuvre "CleftCraft," a very original title for a medical textbook.

The residents. Les Hovey was my chief. Les had been an Army doctor before Miami and went on to be part of the Stanford program. After him was Gene Tanski. Then me, then Gary Burget, who had a special relationship with Walter Garst, who helped him with many nasal reconstructions. Then Mal Lesavoy, who ended up at UCLA, then Bill Riley, Bill Little (who had already finished a residency at Case Western), Scott Spear, Larry Ketch, Leo McCafferty, who all went on to take leadership roles in plastic surgery. Chairman of the RRC, Chairman of ABPS (2), President ASPRS, President ASMS, Founding Member ISCFS, and he ended with Aly Ali, who became the leader in post-bariatric surgery rehabilitation.

Millard's contributions.

Millard was unique in the US since he was a leader in reconstructive surgery as well as maintaining a busy aesthetic practice. The waiting period for a Millard facelift was 2 years, and I received many referrals from Millard for patients who didn't want to wait that long.

He was the universally acknowledged expert on cleft lip, with 80% of cleft surgeons worldwide using the rotation advancement, or Millard repair.

In aesthetic surgery he was one of the first to include the neck in a facelift, in a paper coauthored with Walter Garst.

Reed Dingman and other noted plastic surgeons brought their wives to him, as did Jack Anderson, the founder of the Facial Plastic Group.

He was the acknowledged leader in secondary rhinoplasty.

In spite of, perhaps because of, the acceptance that he was the best American plastic surgeon, there was jealousy, the opponents to his becoming President of ASPRS resorted to chicanery to keep him out of the position. He was blackballed from the Association. Millard was not a gregarious person, and was ill at ease at cocktail parties. Besides his wife Barbara, he did not have many close friends.

With the residents and fellows, he was continually asking "What's the principle here?" and he went on to expand on the principles espoused in Gillies and Millard, which ended up with the publication of another book with a clever title, "The Principalization of Plastic Surgery." What the residents learned from him was attention to fine detail and were asked to define the "ideal beautiful norm." One year we had a resident named Norm who of course became The Ideal Beautiful Norm.

Millard had a close relationship with most of his residents, who in spite of being banged on during the residency, in most cases appreciated the close scrutiny and the teaching.

After I became his associate, I had a frosty relationship with Millard, there would be a shadow in my doorway, and Millard would say, "This isn't working out." I would respond "Why?" He would then say that I had bought my secretary a new rug or typewriter, and now his wanted one. Finally, he did it again and I said, "Dr. Millard, bullshit." He recoiled slightly but left me alone from then on.

I was touched when long after his death, I noticed the inscription he wrote for my copy of Principalization in 1987. "To Tony, Thanks for your contributions in this book and for the years of working together. Great years!"

When he was President of AAPS at the Coronado meeting he asked me to be the Program Chairman. He devoted his Presidential address to Principles, and gave an example for each one.

The whole focus on Principles I am sure Millard got from Sir Harold Gillies, who listed in his 1920 book, Plastic Surgery of the Face a number, ("replace like tissue with like", "put things in their normal position and keep them there") which were added to in Gillies and Millard (now a total of ten, and even more in Principalization. (Up to 33)

Harry Buncke certainly deserves credit for popularizing microsurgery and free tissue transfer (which Millard criticized for being nothing but "O-filling" without any concern for the final aesthetic result).

But Millard deserves being ranked as the top plastic surgeon of the 20th century in my opinion.

What did I learn from him?

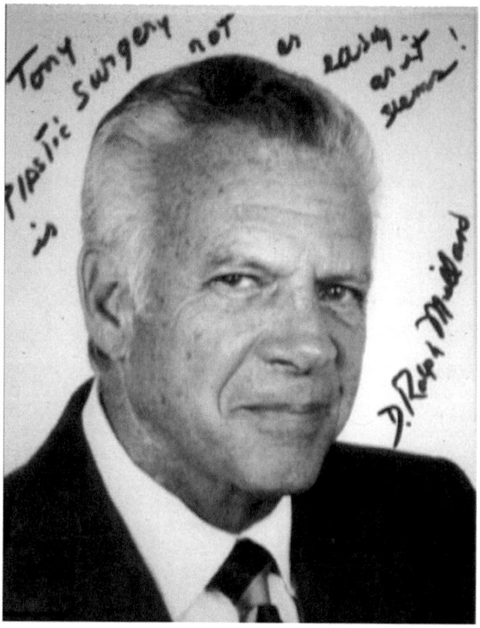
Tony
Plastic surgery is not as easy as it seems!
D. Ralph Millard

1. Attention to fine detail. Being able to convince the patient to have one more minor procedure.
2. Respect for facial aesthetic units.
3. Proper documentation with good photography. Evy Dyer was our photographer for years, followed by George Insua who is still with us. Evy was also a fine medical artist and did the drawings for my book.
4. **The rotation advancement for unilateral clefts**. And although Millard felt I was disloyal in not using the forked flap for columellar lengthening, (the staged rotation-advancements providing perfectly normal collumellas). I am sure that after his initial complaints that he would quietly adopt the procedure and probably improve upon it.
5. How to make and transfer a tube pedicle—not difficult.

Preparations for Paris

I was able to cobble together a number of small scholarships, including one from The International College of Surgeons. Walter Garst provided some support and eventually I was able to get a Bourse from the French Government, similar to a Fulbright, and all told it was enough to modestly live on.

Later in the year, when I was a regular assistant, Tessier would from time to time give me a check on an American bank.

Vladimir Mitz was spending time with Millard, so we switched dwellings, the Erikson guest house for his Paris apartment. I went from there to 5 or 6 different places, ending up on the 7th floor of a building on rue Boileau, where a demented lady in an adjacent apartment would scream at night. The police would come but there was nothing they could do about it.

Clinique Belvédere

Tessier did 90% of his work at Belvedere, which was originally an obstetrical hospital where European Royalty would come for their *accoouchements*.

It had three operating rooms in the basement plus another small room for dressing changes. Often he occupied all three operating rooms: one case being put to sleep, one being operated upon, and in the third the assistants would be suturing a completed case.

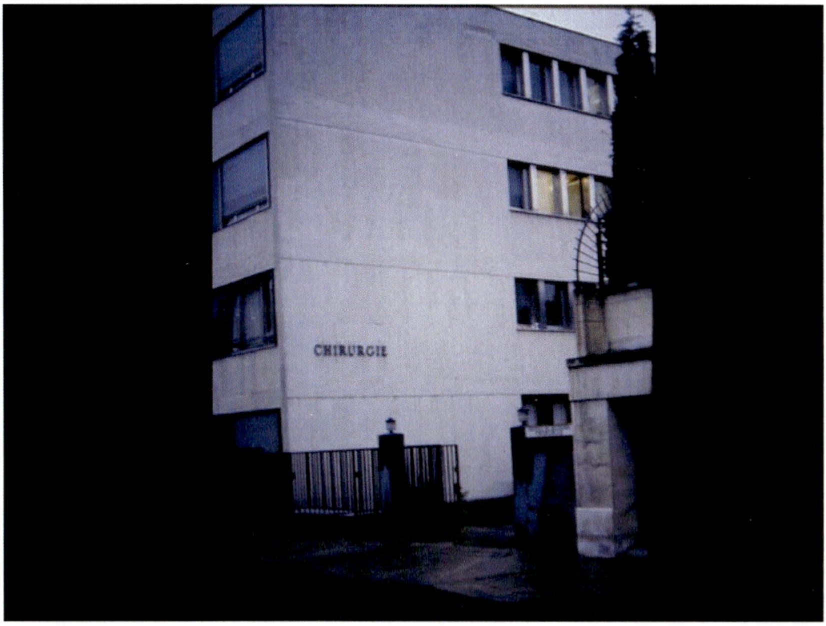

Clinique Belvedere

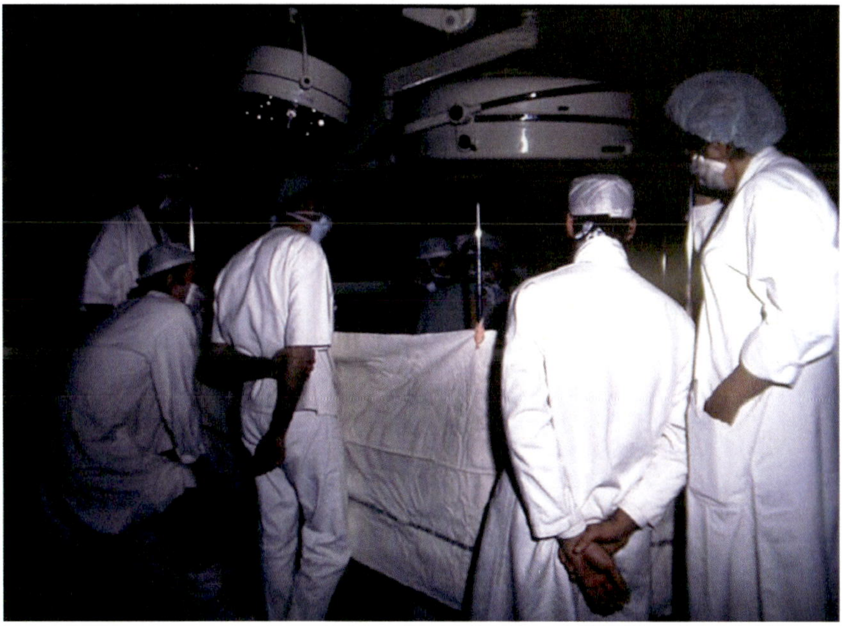

The sheet between two IV poles as a barrier.

One afternoon a week he went to Hôspital Foch to run a small clinic and then operate, often finishing close to midnight. He had done his early craniofacial cases at Foch, including the first transcranial case with neurosurgeon Gerard Guiot (Bernadette Le Roy), but took most of his practice to Belvedere after repeated complaints from the anesthesia and nursing staffs about working so late.

At Belvedere, all of the staff - nurses, scrub nurses, orderlies, anesthesiologists - worked for Tessier, so he could work as long as he wanted and organize everything to his liking.

I arrived at Belvedere in July of 1974, not knowing where to go.

The Morrocan orderly, Idir, gave me a scrub suit and I went back to the OR where Tessier was involved in a case. There were at least a dozen onlookers behind a sheet stretched between two IV poles to keep the crowd at a distance.

The onlookers thinned out as the evening went on, and by 8:00 there were no visitors other than me, with three operation to go, finishing at midnight. I finally introduced myself and said I was from Millard. Ah, he said, "how is Ralph?" I think Tessier enjoyed these late night conversations we had which covered a wide range of topics, including *contrepeteries* - spoonerisms. This may explain his large use of acronyms like S.M.A.S.

Millard would do two to three cases a day, with a leisurely turnover time, and leave in the early afternoon.

Tessier would do 10 to 15 cases a day, with no turnover time, and leave at 11:30 at night, six days a week, with Saturday being the busiest day.

Half of the schedule was garden variety plastic surgery, facelifts, eyelids, breast reduction (very rarely an augmentation, and a very small volume of 150 to 200 cc), abdominoplasties - but the other half was bone surgery: bone grafts to the orbit, maxillary osteotomies, and intracranial procedures. It was thrilling to see the precision of the bone carpentry and the harvesting and use of bone grafts—mostly iliac, some rib. I had never seen bone surgery performed so precisely, mostly through a coronal incision, which I had not seen in Miami.

During the day, I was one of the onlookers behind the sheet, and I continued to stay on as often the sole audience as Tessier operated until the late evening. Finally, after about 3 weeks, Elizabeth Hecht, Tessier's scrub nurse indicated to me that I should scrub. I think it was a facelift—familiar territory—and I was tasked with suturing the incisions. This was a test of my suturing skills.

I must have passed muster since I now belonged to the assistants' pool. That was a step up from being behind the IV poles, but the bad thing would be that I would be sewing up a facelift or breast reduction while a Crouzon or hypertelorism was being done in the next room, that I really wanted to see. I gradually became part of the A-team, and Dr. Tessier would from time to time give me a check from an American patient.

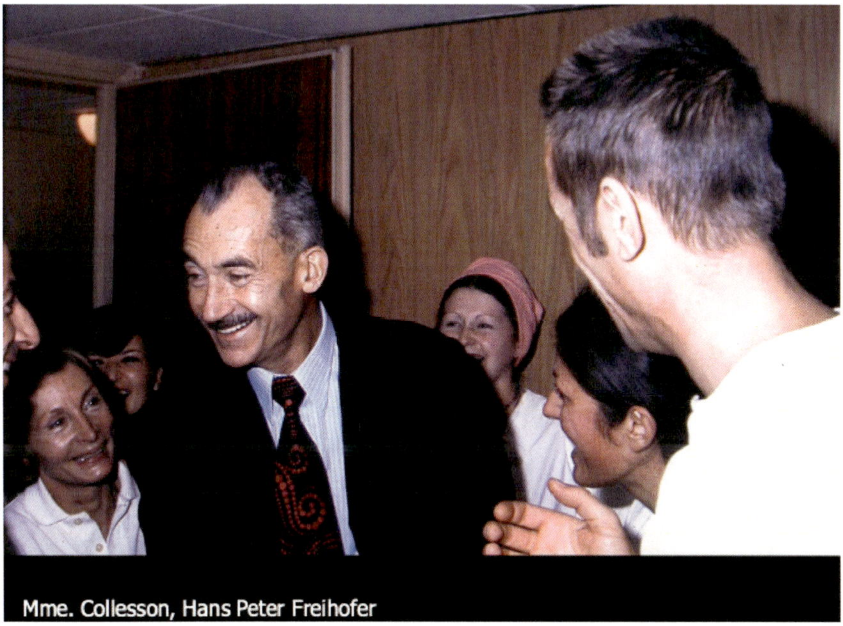

Tessier at graduation party for Yvon Raulo, who had been his assistant and was in the office with him for several years. Andree Collesson, anesthetist to his right, Hans Peter Freihofer from Obwegeser in Zurich who had been Tessier's first foreign Fellow, Elizabeth Hecht, scrub nurse between the two.

I had little time to explore Paris with the 15-hour days at the clinic and sometimes Foch. Dr. Tessier would go to Iran every few months for a few weeks, and that time gave an opportunity to visit - at Tessier's suggestion—with Jacques Dautrey, a true master of the sagittal split. I also went to Zurich to visit Obwegeser's unit and graciously he did not charge me the usual visitors fee.

Completing training in Paris

Midway in my year in Paris, there was a meeting in Chicago, one of the first on Craniofacial Surgery, staged by Sam Pruzansky, an orthodontist who had been Berkowitz's teacher. I traveled with the team, and met Henry Kawamoto, a Converse trainee who was at UCLA, who had been with Tessier for 6 months and who left Paris just before my arrival. Henry and I became fast friends. Aside from that, there was a period of several weeks available while Tessier went each year to the Central African Republic to hunt elephants.

The year went by quickly and my last day arrived. There was a going away party for me, and I was given a copy of Tord Skoog's book inscribed by everyone. I had had a fabulous year, but now it was time to return to Miami. What had I learned from Tessier?

The importance of wide subperiosteal dissection to expose the facial skeleton.

The importance of good power equipment, instrumentation, and surgical syringes. I bought $70,000 worth of instruments from French, Swedish, and German companies. I was able to buy Heljestrand osteotomes, which Tessier said were the best, but alas, the company no longer exists.

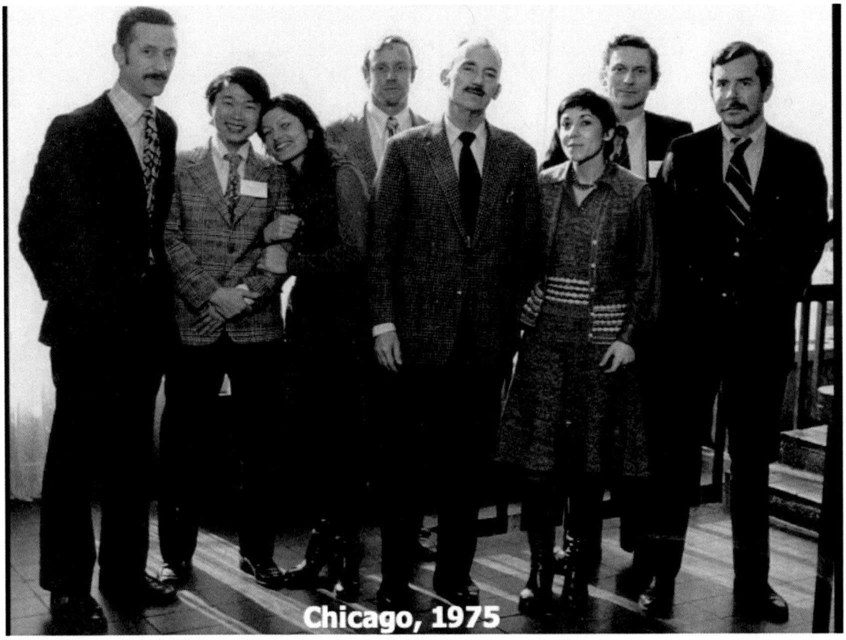

One of the first meetings dedicated entirely to Craniofacial Surgery was put on in Chicago in 1975 by the head of the CCFA (Center for Craniofacial Anomalies at The University of Illinois) Sam Pruzansky. From left: Hans Peter, Henry Kawamoto, Elizabeth Hecht, Doug Ousterhaut, PLT, Martine Peyronie, Walter Pepersack, SAW. (There was another meeting in Chicago 20 years later, in Dr. Tessier's honor, organized by Joe McCarthy of NYU.)

At the meeting there was a dinner in a Club to which those who had been close to Dr. Tessier were invited. Milton Edgerton had never visited Tessier or seen him operate in the US, but he got Joe Murray to include him. After dinner there were remarks given, and Edgerton rose to speak. He praised Tessier, but said that he had had the idea for hypertelorism correction and the Le Fort 3 independently, and was unaware of Tessier's work when he did his first cases.

This was false: I recalled what he had told me during my residency interview. After dinner I accosted Edgerton and heatedly and impolitely said that what he had claimed was untrue, and asked why, of all the Founding Members of ISCFS he was the only one who never visited Tessier. I didn't get an answer.

Years later I was visiting a professor at the University of Virginia, where Edgerton was now Chief after leaving Hopkins. At the dinner he was charming and friendly to my daughter Olivia who had come with me, more of a gentleman than I had been. Not a word was said about the episode in Chicago.

Here are a few of Tessier's iconic cases shown in Chicago in 1975 and 1995:

Burgaud, a 0-14 cleft, with a result that could not be obtained by any contemporary surgeon - this over 50 years ago!

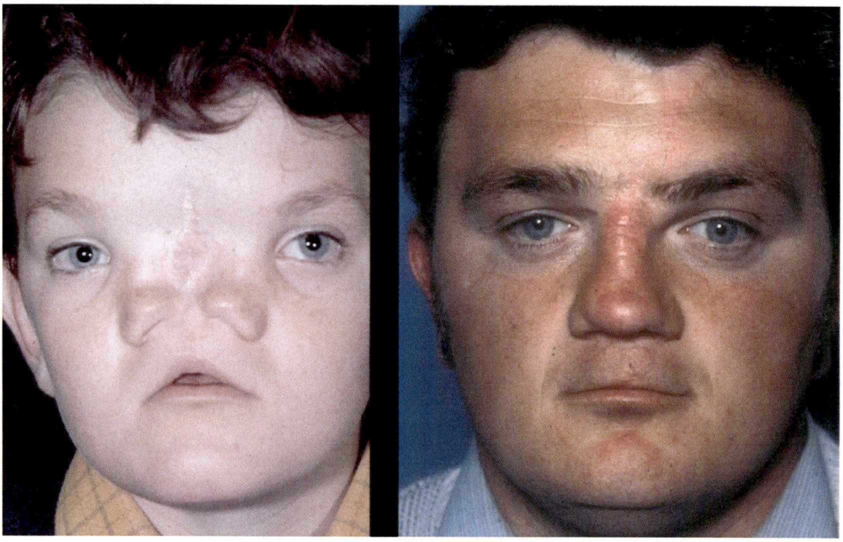

Bourgaud.

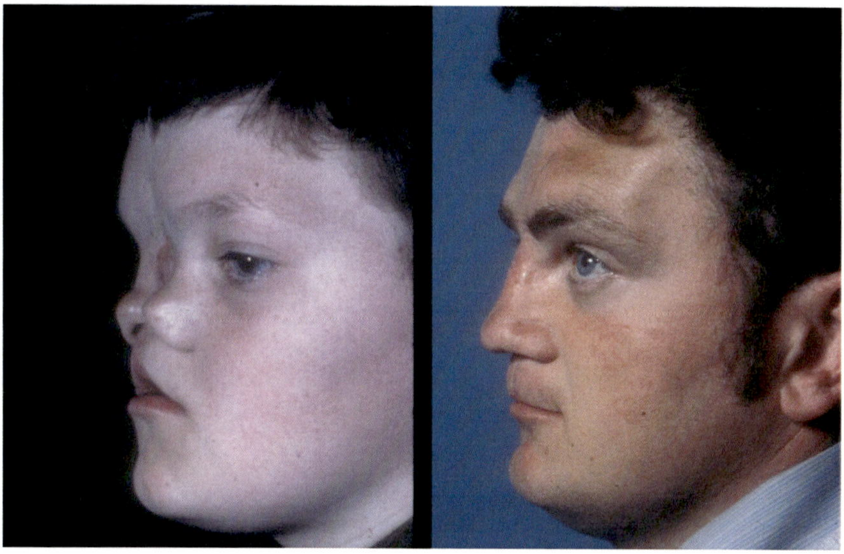

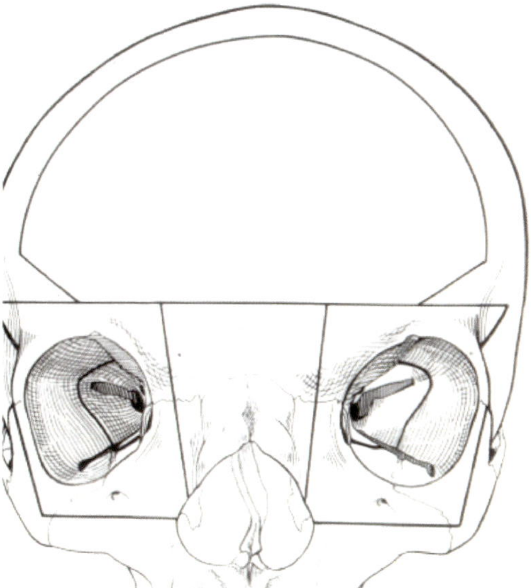

In Europe the left side is generally shown for the lateral view; in the US, it is the right.

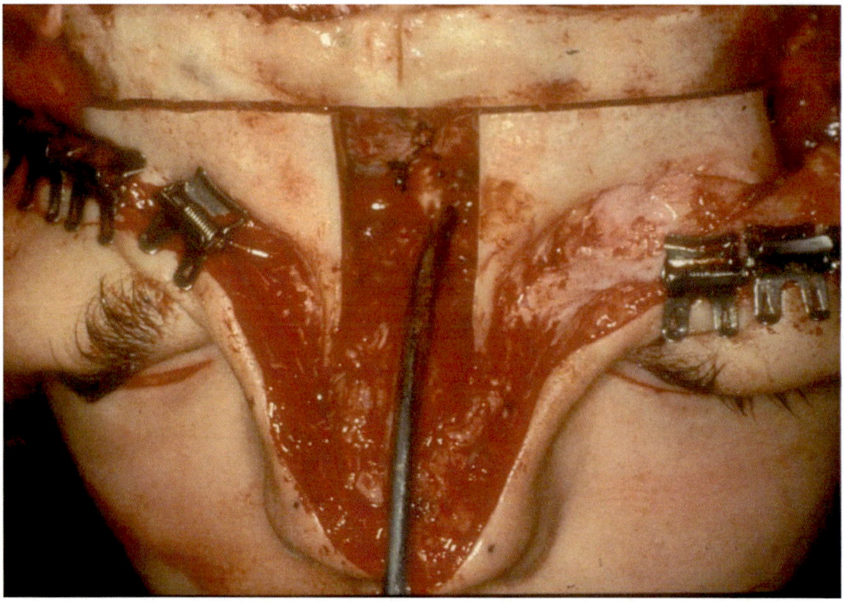

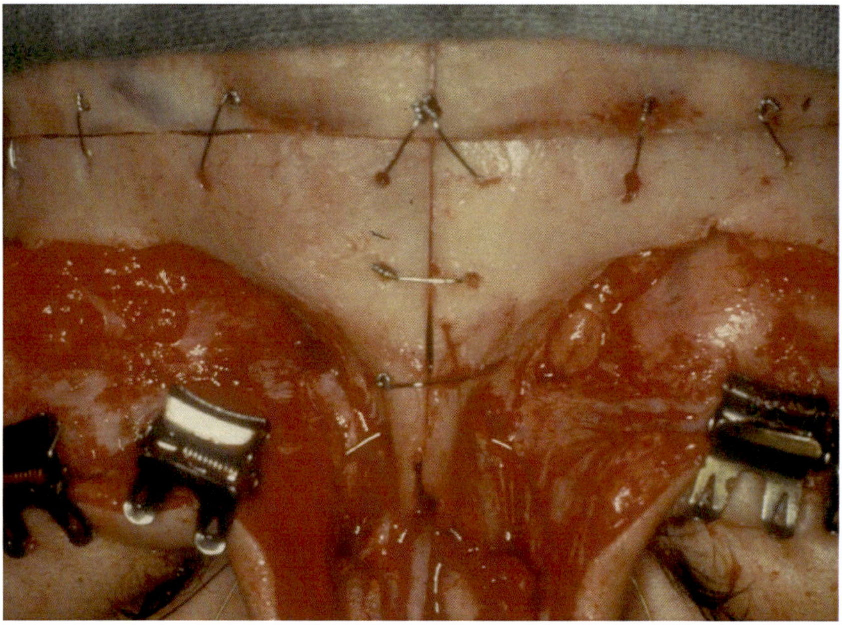

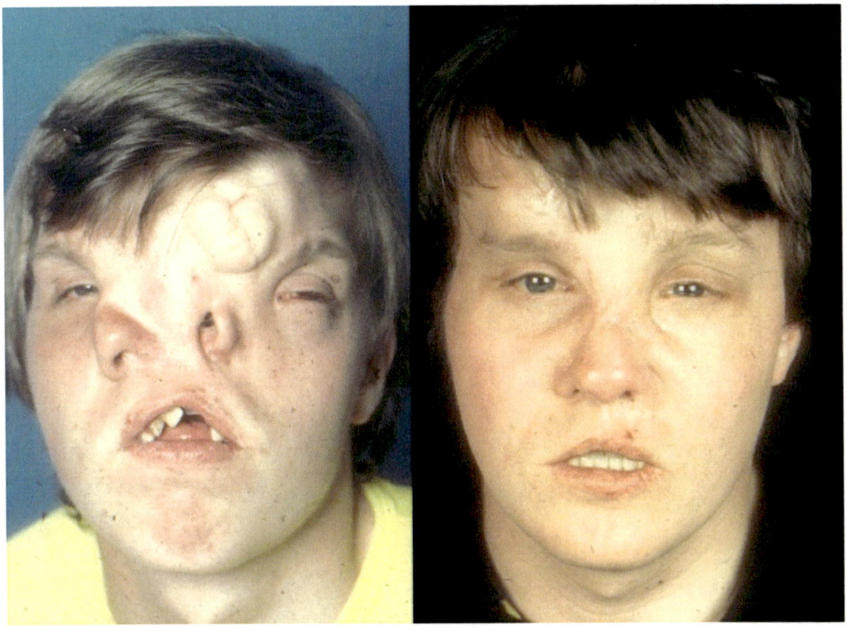

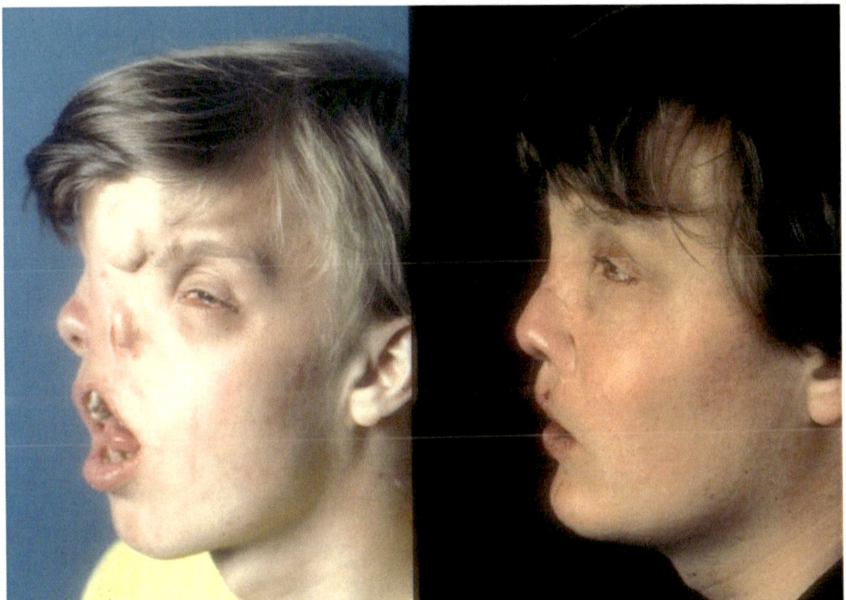

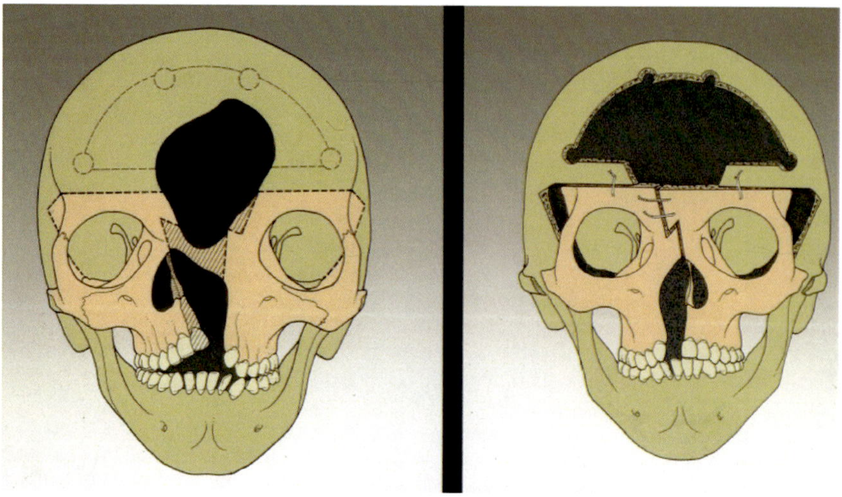

Complex facial bipartition with interlocking bone fixation.

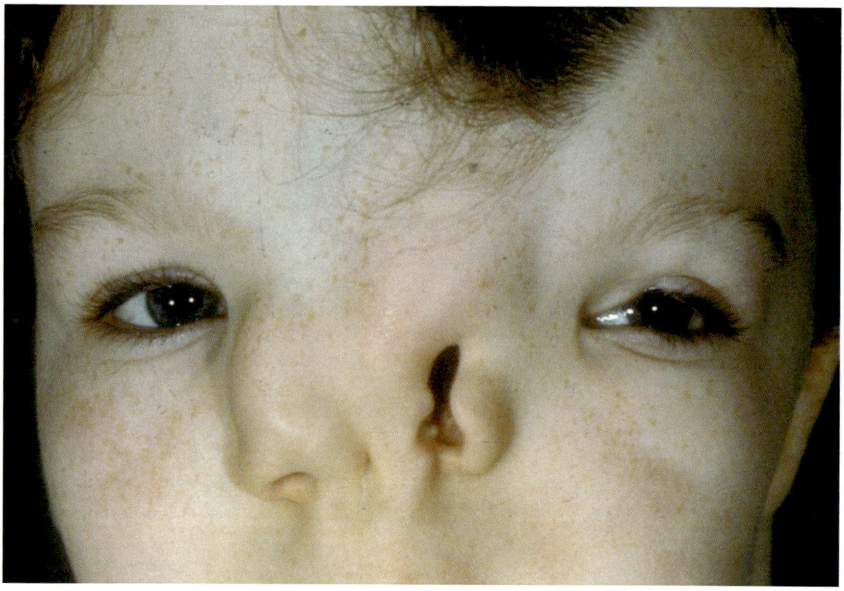

Multiple facial clefts and wide hypertelorism, nasal clefting.

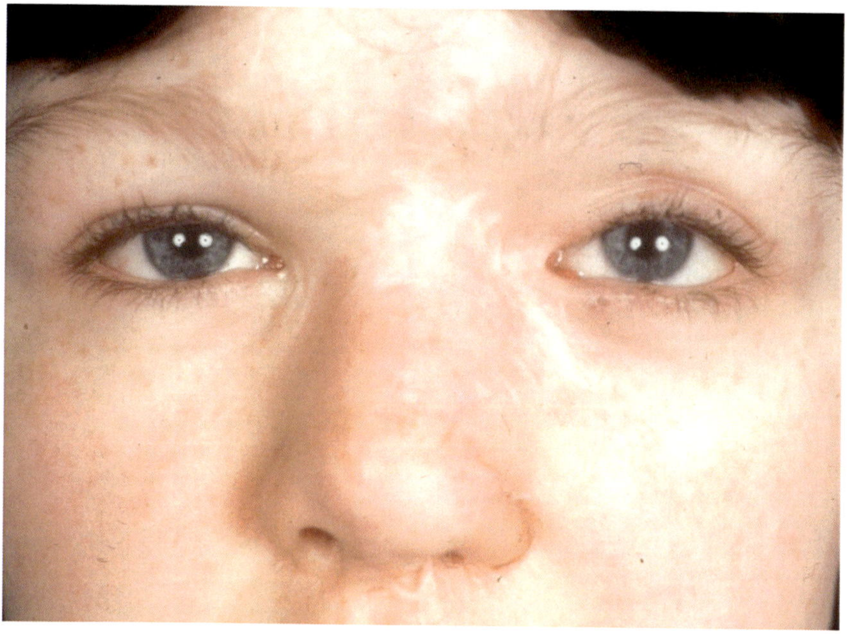

These Tessier hypertelorism cases are unmatched. No one since has achieved results of this quality.

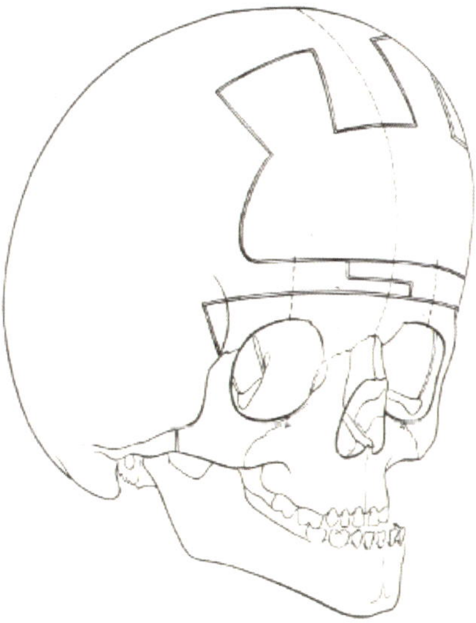

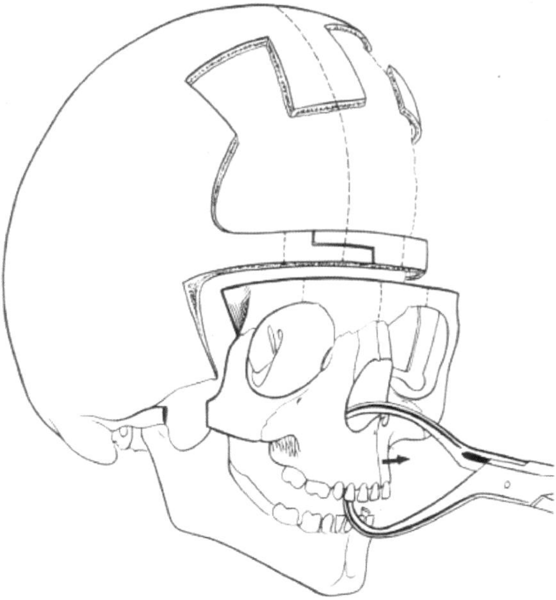

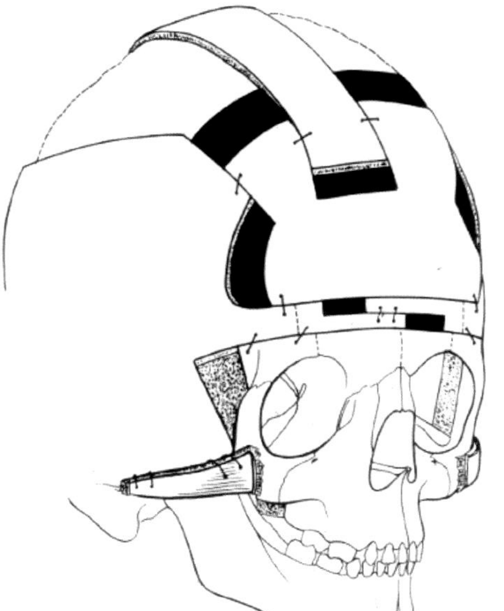

Here are two Tessier cases who were treated with a monobloc (advancement of forehead, orbits and midface) frontofacial advancement (MFFA). The remarkable thing is that this was before the introduction of titanium plates and screws - he had only wire to stabilize the bone segments.

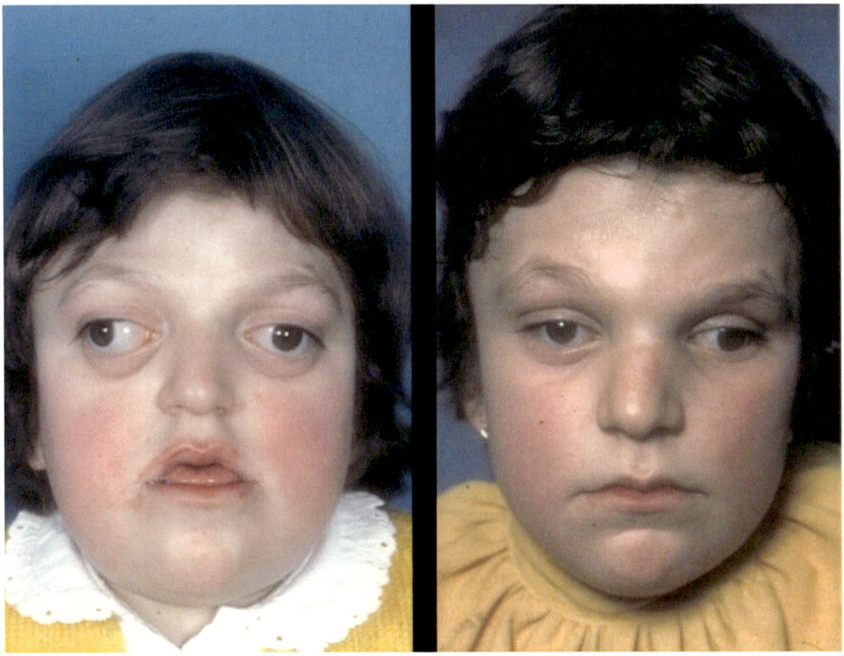

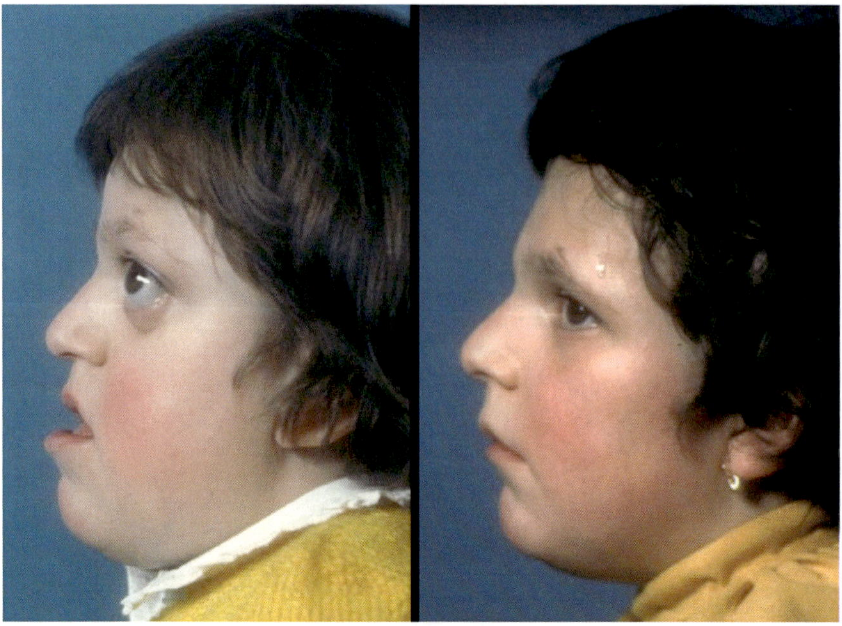

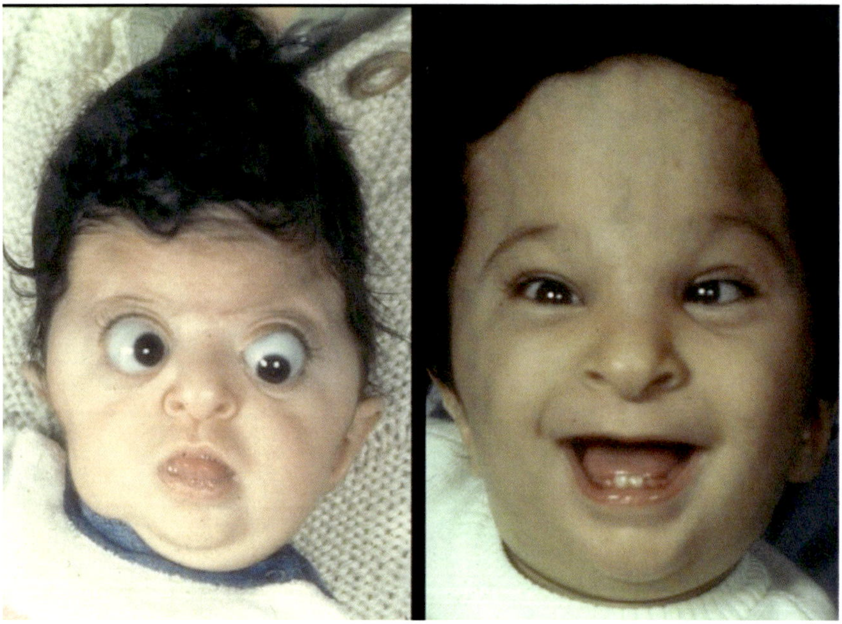

Here is a case of mine, done with rigid plate and screw fixation, but without distraction. For milder cases distraction is not necessary surgeons use it for all cases, but there is often some distortion of the lateral canthus.

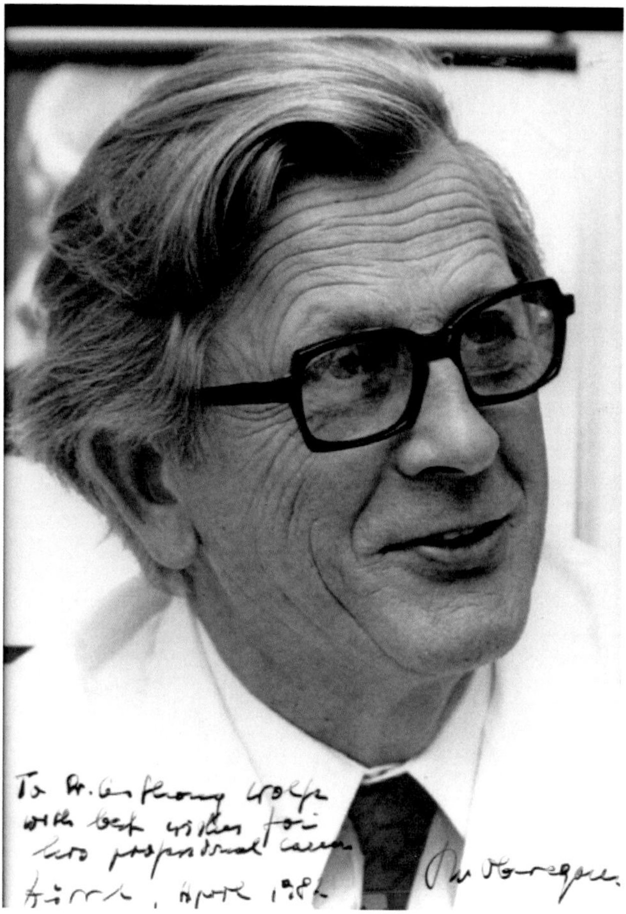

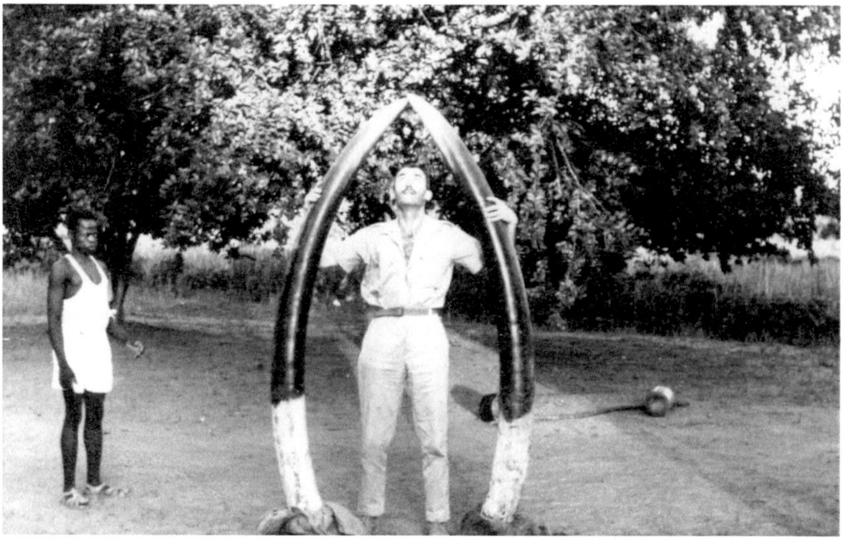

Tessier with horns of his elephant, circa 1965.

The year went by quickly and my last day arrived. There was a going away party for me, and I was given a copy of Tord Skoog's book with inscriptions from the entire staff.

Tessier's inscription, at the bottom of the page, reads, "And now sow the grain and make it grow well and we will reap the harvest in ten years."

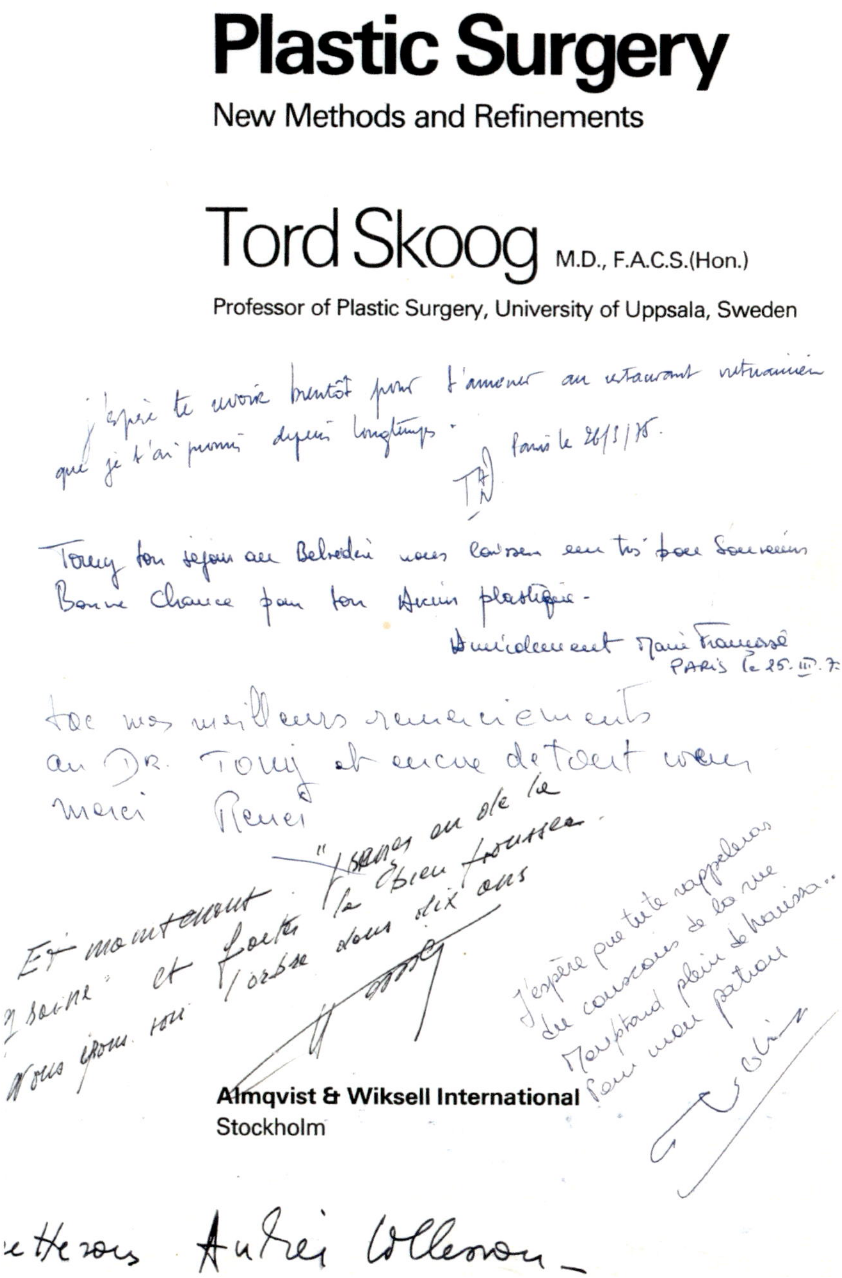

Plastic Surgery

New Methods and Refinements

Tord Skoog M.D., F.A.C.S.(Hon.)

Professor of Plastic Surgery, University of Uppsala, Sweden

Almqvist & Wiksell International
Stockholm

Inscribed by everyone. I had had a fabulous year, but now it was time to return to Miami. What had I learned from Tessier?

1. The importance of wide subperiosteal dissection to expose the facial skeleton.
2. The importance of good power equipment and instrumentation, and surgical syringes. I bought $70,000 worth of instruments from French, Swedish, and German companies. I was able to buy Heljestrand osteotomes, which Tessier said was the best steel. They lasted my entire career. The best wire was French, from the Societe des Cendres. Like Heljestrand, the Societe de Cendres is out of business. Getting good wire proved to be a constant problem. American wire was too brittle, the Aesculap Company had good wire available, but they would not export it to the US. I had a friend in Italy buy it, but that was a challenge too.
3. The importance of rigid fixation, wire or increasingly plates and screws (Champys, stainless steel, then Luhr titanium).
4. The vital importance of good power equipment - Tessier at first had only a Stryker cast cutter—a large oscillating saw. The next improvement was the Stryker air driven equipment, which was the first one I used in Miami. It also had a drill and reciprocating saw. A year later when I was visiting Tessier in Paris (as I did most years) I noticed a strange piece of equipment which had arms and a cloth shield, somewhat like a sail. This was the Aesculap, a fine power tool with an electric motor, I bought the first one to be sold in the US, and was asked to speak to their sales force at their headquarters in Burlingame, near the San Francisco airport.
5. But more important than the equipment were the ideas, the principles, the logic of the work: the concept of the effective orbit, that segment of the orbital framework which when moved takes the globe with it, making possible the correction of vertical and horizontal orbital dystopias, the classification of clefts (later to become clefts and agenesis), the forward movement of the midface by Le Fort 1 and 3 osteotomies and the

monobloc fronto facial advancement, the use of the temporal muscle in many areas in the face including septation of the cranial base from the face, and maxillary reconstruction.

6. An understanding of skeletal anatomy, both normal and abnormal. One cannot provide a definitive correction of a condition without knowing what is missing or displaced.

Tessier's training

Tessier's father, Ernest, suffered shell shock in WW1, and was captured by the Germans. At the time, the belligerent countries had an understanding that prisoners of war could be shipped to a neutral country as long as they agreed not to rejoin their comrades at arms. The elder Tessier was sent to a camp in Switzerland where conjugal visits were permitted, so it is likely that Paul Tessier was conceived in Switzerland.

After the war Ernest remained a semi-invalid, and the younger Tessier was raised by his maternal grandfather Auguste Clergeau, a wine retailer. Paul had his schooling in Heric, and went on to medical school in Nantes in 1936. He was mobilized into the army in 1938, and was confined to his hospital, Hotel Dieu after the German blitzkrieg. In 1941 Tessier became quite ill—febrile and comatose. He was transferred to a German military hospital, where no diagnosis could be made. Finally, his Professor of Medicine was allowed to see him, and immediately diagnoses typhoid fever.

The American Airforce bombed Nantes in 1943, completely destroying Hotel Dieu, so Tessier got to Paris, by hitchhiking and bicycle. In Paris, he was able to find employ with Maurice Virenque, who had a position as maxillofacial surgeon at Hôspital Foch. Tessier also worked with George Huc, a pediatric surgeon that he greatly admired. Tessier had a particularly close relationship with the Sourdille family, father and son ophthalmologists in Nantes, and he had many referrals from ophthalmologists, including Lille, where he went several times a year to operate on orbital and eyelid cases.

In the decade following the end of WW2 Tessier did a very large amount of facial reconstructive surgery on those wounded in the war, both military and civilian. Plastic surgery did not exist in France as a separate specialty even though Hippolyte Morestin was a pioneer in the early days of WW1 and was responsible for Harold Gillies to begin reconstruction for the facial injuries that were so common in this fox hole war. Tessier had a broad training in facial surgery, working as an assistant to a maxillofacial, pediatric and ENT surgeon.

Between 1946 and 1950 Tessier made 6 trips of 1-2 months visiting plastic units in Great Britain, Archibald MacIndoe in particular, but also to Sir Harold Gillies.

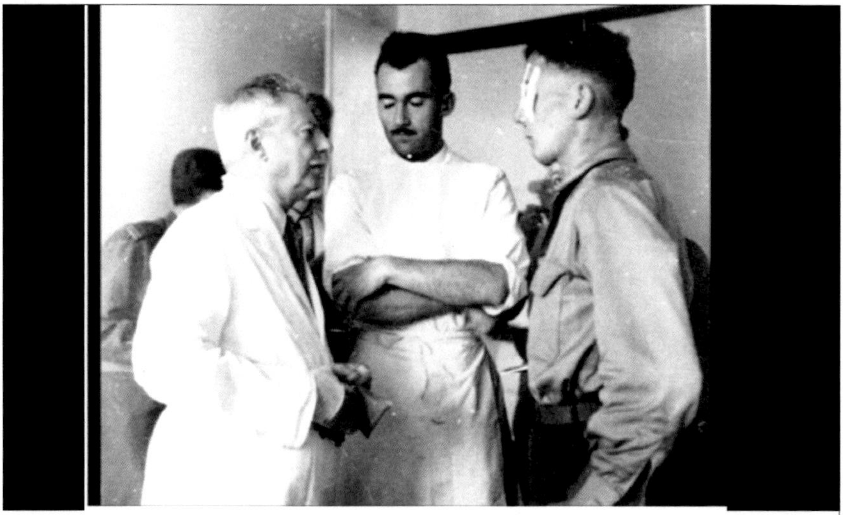

Maurice Virenque and Paul Tessier, 1954, Paris, examining a wounded soldier (Brother of Jacques Dautrey, a superb maxillofacial surgeon who later collaborated with Tessier at Hopital Foch

Tessier served on the service of Maurice Virenque at Hôspital Foch. He also had a position running the burn unit, and the quality of his burn reconstructions remains unrivalled to the present day.

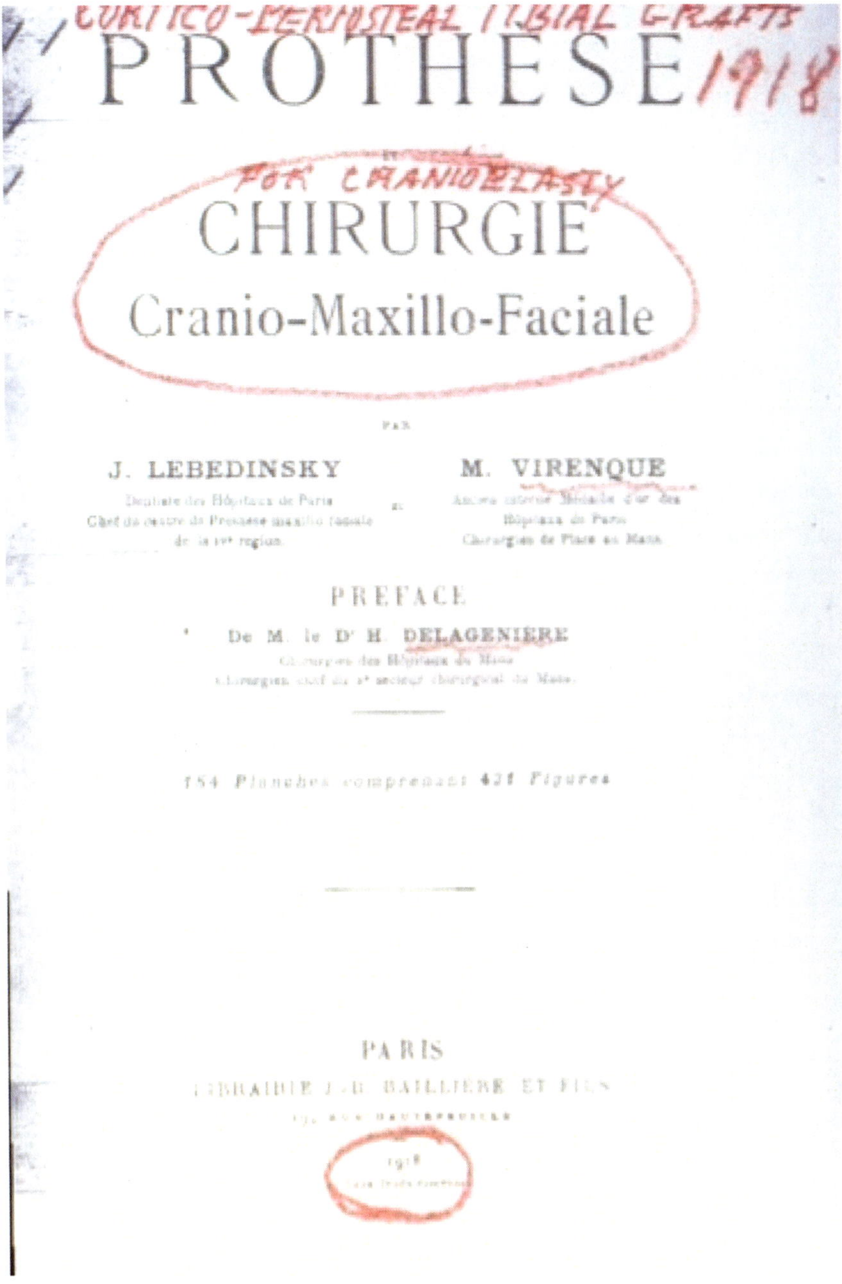

Tessier's copy of Virenque's 1918 book. The term Cranio-maxillo-facial is nothing new.

In the 1950's and 1960's he extended his horizon to North and South America, making a trip in 1951 that lasted 5 months, visiting Jerome Webster in New York, Sterling Bunnell in San Francisco, James Barret Brown and others of his service in St. Louis. On subsequent trips he visited Ralph Millard, Mario Gonzales-Ulloa, and Fernando Ortiz-Monasterio (who remained a lifelong friend).

In the decade of the 1950's he had visited every major plastic surgeon in the world. Tessier was an autodidact, putting together his own training with time spent working with pediatric surgeons, ENT, orthopods, and eventually neurosurgeons in France, and adding to it, knowledge gleaned from his international travels.

Tessier's work with burns is often overlooked because of his creation of the field of craniofacial surgery. In this patient he obtained an outstanding result, including eyebrow and even eyelash grafts. In the other he did outstanding eyelid grafting as well as a total nasal reconstruction.

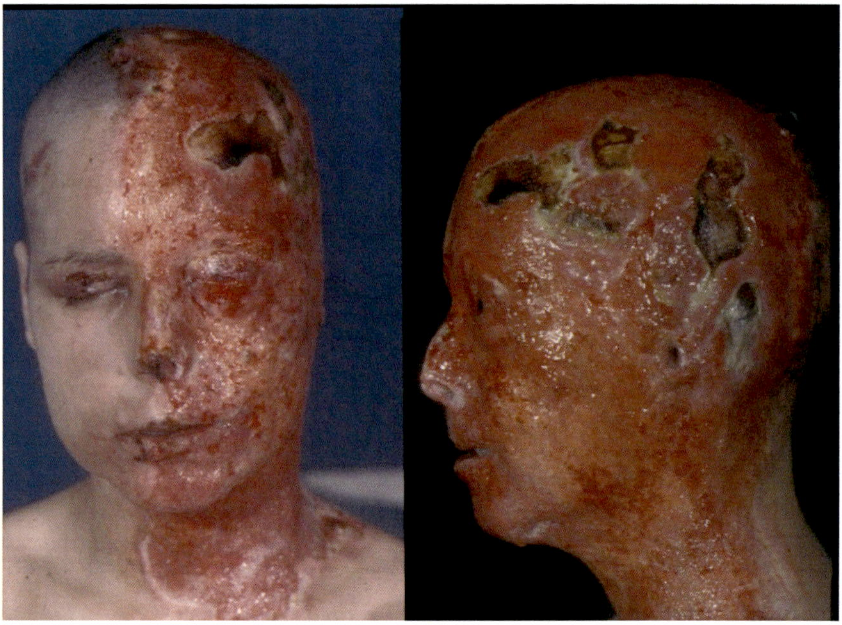

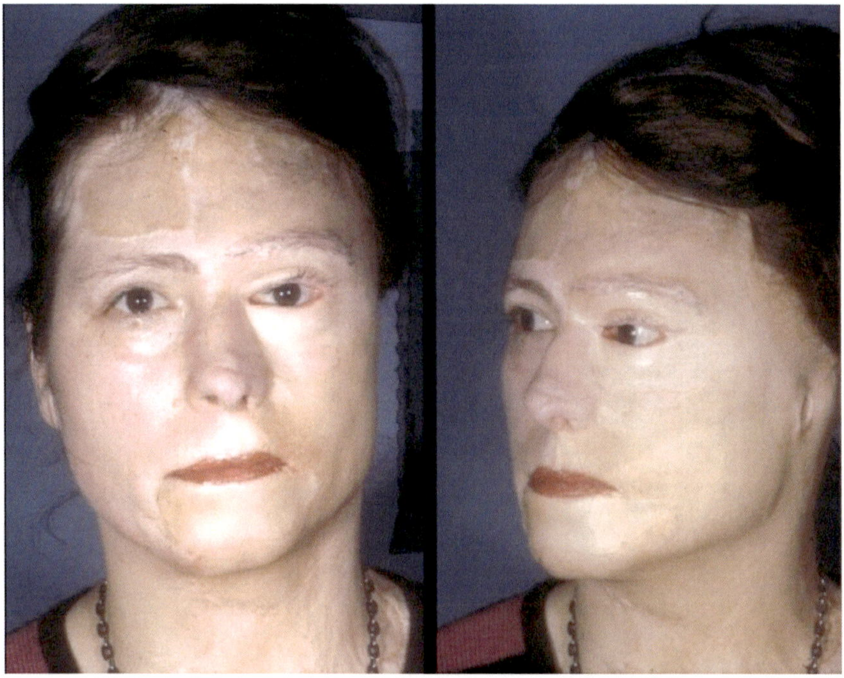

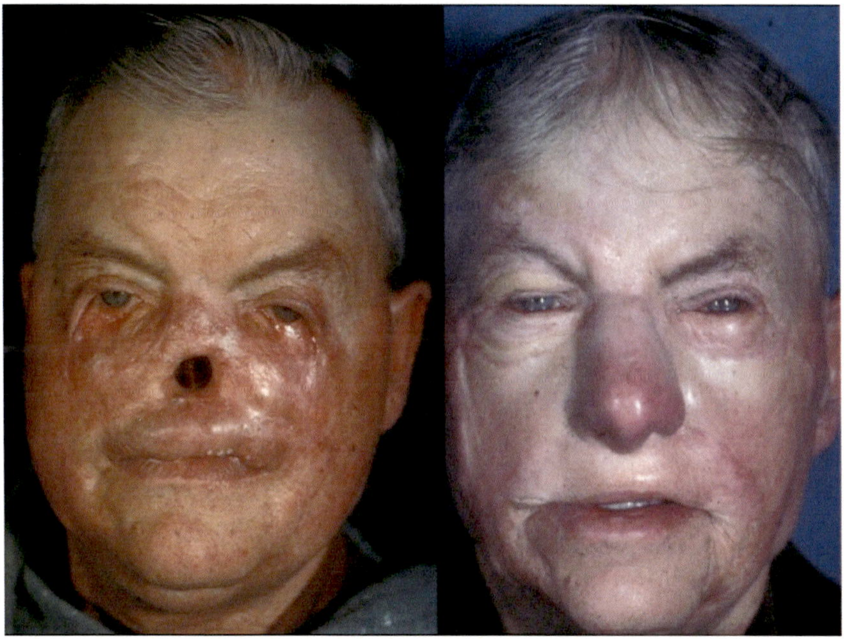

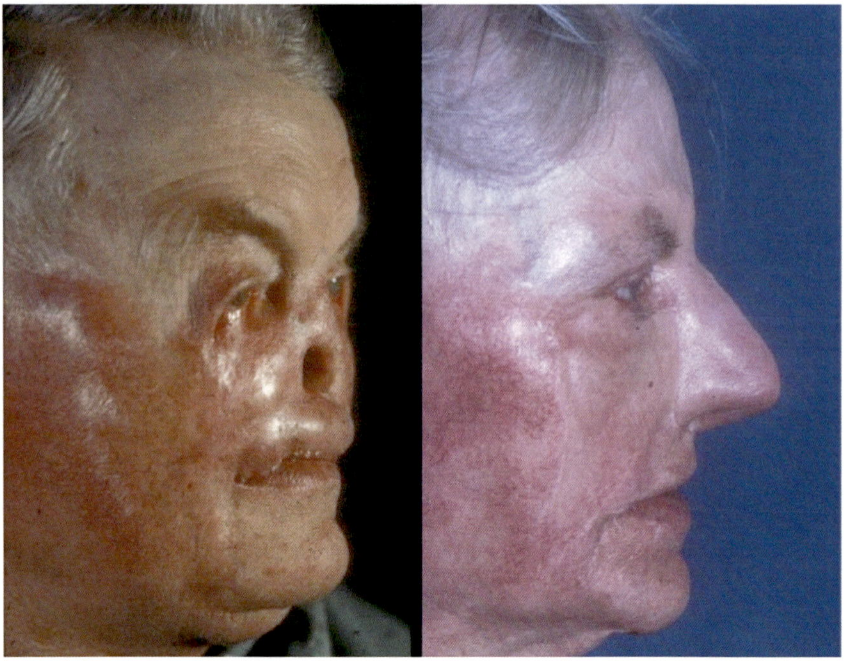

Ginestet

Gustave Ginestet ran the other maxillofacial service at Foch, and after the death (by suicide) of Virenque, Tessier had lost his Patron.

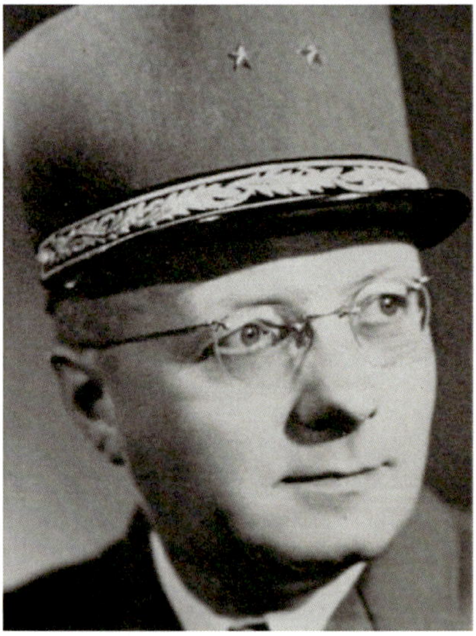

Tessier received the following letter from Ginestet in 1962.

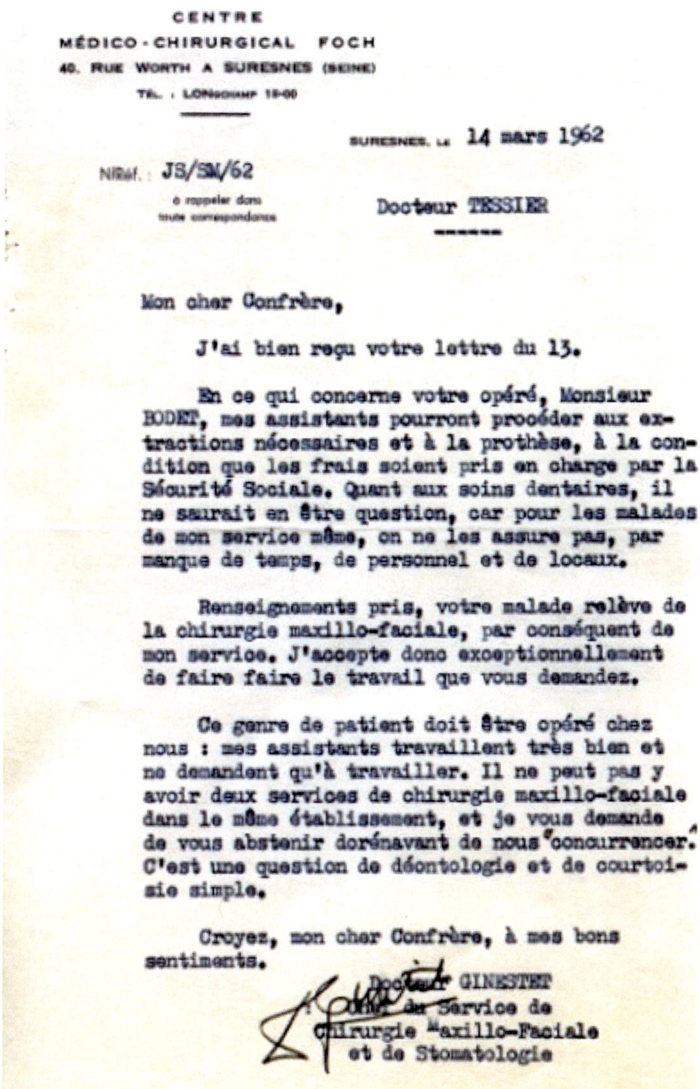

CENTRE
MÉDICO-CHIRURGICAL FOCH
40, RUE WORTH A SURESNES (SEINE)
TÉL. : LONGCHAMP 19-00

SURESNES, LE 14 mars 1962

N/Réf. : JS/SM/62
à rappeler dans toute correspondance

Docteur TESSIER

Mon cher Confrère,

J'ai bien reçu votre lettre du 13.

En ce qui concerne votre opéré, Monsieur BODET, mes assistants pourront procéder aux extractions nécessaires et à la prothèse, à la condition que les frais soient pris en charge par la Sécurité Sociale. Quant aux soins dentaires, il ne saurait en être question, car pour les malades de mon service même, on ne les assure pas, par manque de temps, de personnel et de locaux.

Renseignements pris, votre malade relève de la chirurgie maxillo-faciale, par conséquent de mon service. J'accepte donc exceptionnellement de faire faire le travail que vous demandez.

Ce genre de patient doit être opéré chez nous : mes assistants travaillent très bien et ne demandent qu'à travailler. Il ne peut pas y avoir deux services de chirurgie maxillo-faciale dans le même établissement, et je vous demande de vous abstenir dorénavant de nous "concurrencer." C'est une question de déontologie et de courtoisie simple.

Croyez, mon cher Confrère, à mes bons sentiments.

Docteur GINESTET
Chef du Service de
Chirurgie Maxillo-Faciale
et de Stomatologie

Ginestet is telling Tessier that there cannot be two maxillofacial services in the same establishment and demands that he stop "competing with us" and stick to the treatment of burns.

Fortunately for the sake of plastic surgery, Tessier ignored Ginestet.

There was no keeping the genie in the bottle. In January of 1958 Tessier saw an unusual patient in named Anquetil.

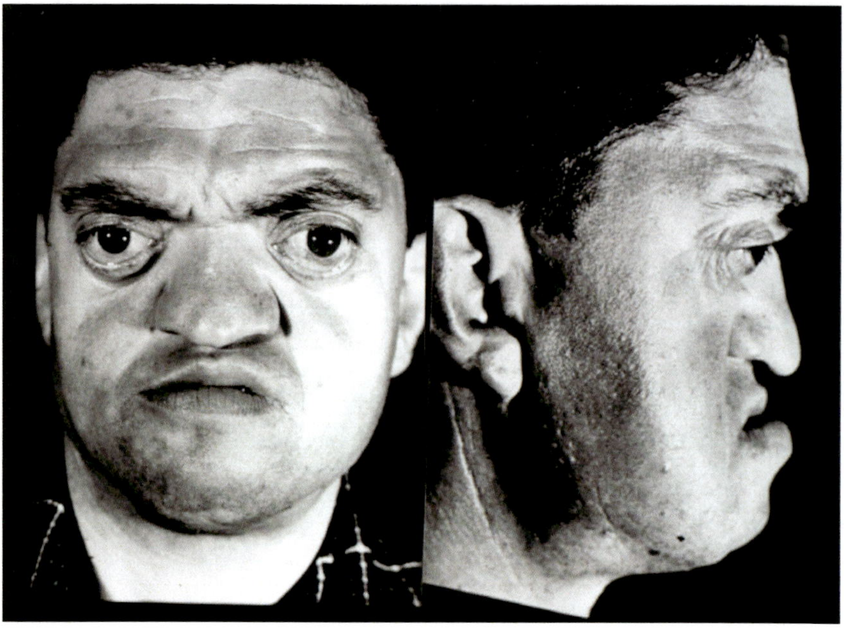

Here is Tessier's note:

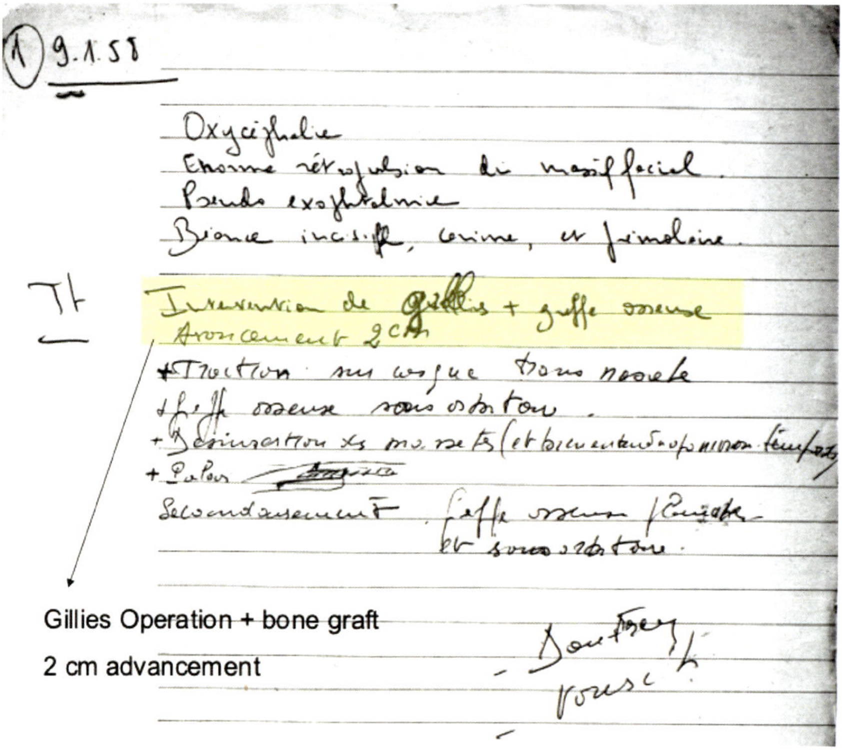

He says the treatment would involve the "Gillies procedure" plus a bone graft.

Nom : ANQUETIL   Sexe : M   Lieu : FOCH

Date : 26.2.1958

CRO.

I – Voie d'abord palatine et interptérygo maxillaire D et G.

a) Incision en U ouvert en AR
La branche transversale du U est à 2 cm en AV du bord postérieur du palais.

Rugination du palais.

Ostéotomie (burin large à nez) palatine transversale à 5 m/m en AV du bord postérieur du palais. Elle doit donc se situer dans la suture maxillo palatine. Elle va d'un trou palatin à l'autre.

b) Les branches sagittales du U contournent en dedans le trou palatin et en AR l'arcade dentaire.

Ostéotomie interptérygo maxillaire (burins larges et courbes; rugines "dites américaines" aiguisées)

Cette ostéotomie atteint 2 cm de profondeur et se dirige franchement en dehors.

Difficultés, Dangers, Critiques.

- La fibro muqueuse palatine flotte en drapeau.
- Epargner la palatine postérieure dont les anastomoses avec la palatine antérieure sont une sécurité pour le maxillaire supérieur.
- Toutefois, dans ce cas on sectionne ses branches destinées au voile et cette section peut devenir responsable d'une nécrose du lambeau palatin.
- Epargner la palatine dans son trajet vertical au cours de l'ostéotomie (rester postérieur)

Obtenir une ouverture suffisante de la bouche. L'écarteur de Bott n'est pas valable (rétrogénie)

2 – Voie d'abord zygomatique D et G.

Incision oblique de 10 m/m en B et en AR sur le versant postérie[ur] de la pommette.

8) Formation d'un lambeau tubulé sous-claviculaire gauche, destiné à fermer la communication oro-nasale.

9) La réduction est maintenue par un blocage inter-maxillaire assuré par les gouttières et les tractions d'abord élastiques puis par fils d'acier.

(K 80 + 40/2)

Difficultés - Dangers.

L'angulaire.

Le peu d'écartement latéral possible.

Les ethmoïdales antérieures (hémostase à la cire)

La poulie du G.O.

Le L.P.E. à ne pas désinsérer.

Le dôme du sac à récliner en bas.

La lame criblée.

7 - Ostéotomie de la cloison.

Par l'ostéotomie fronto-nasale introduire l'ostéotome de Stille de 20 cm/m et faisant levier - provoquer un diastasis F.N.

Ciseaux coudés sur le plat.
Sectionner la cloison jusqu'à l'épine nasale postérieure

8 - Mobilisation.

Retirer le packing nasal et buccal.

Aspirer - Bouche et nez.

Pince de Wolsheim protégée de caoutchouc dans chaque narine et sur le palais.

Mobiliser - tirer dans tous les sens pour faire céder les parties molles.

Hypercorriger.

Difficultés - Dangers.

Le masseter, l'aponévrose temporale.

Les parties molles.

Les pédicules vasculaires et nerveux élongués.

La fracture inter-maxillo-malaire difficile à éviter.

Faut-il embrocher transversalement d'un malaire à l'autre à travers un ~~bord~~ inférieur de l'orbite bien fragile ? Et le sac lacrymal !

..

8)

M. ANQUETIL

Consultation 23.12.1958

La contention est excellente. L'hypercorrection manifeste. Il existe un excellent engrainement. La consolidation parait très avancée. On supprime la contention par fils d'acier.

The first true craniofacial case.

The result with Monsieur Anquetil's case was astounding, but it was an extracranial Le Fort 3 - the highest procedure of maxillofacial surgery. The first truly craniofacial case was a girl from Lille, Bernadette Le Roy, who had a wide hypertelorism due to multiple craniofacial clefts. Tessier realized that the correction of this monstrous deformity would require a transcranial approach to retract the brain and safely perform the orbital osteotomies.

He consulted his colleague at Foch, neurosurgeon Gerard Guiot, and asked him if he would collaborate, breaking a number of neurosurgical taboos. As legend has it, Guiot put his feet up on his desk, thought for a minute, and then said "Porquoi pas?" (Why not?). That has now become the motto of the International Society of Craniofacial Surgery.

*The procedure was done in stages with a preliminary dissection of the anterior cranial base and placement of a dermal graft from the abdomen to cover the dura. Six months later, in November 1961, the second stage was performed.

This first transcranial hypertelorism case had an excellent result.

*The International Society of Craniofacial Surgery was founded in Montreal at the International Plastic Surgery Association in Montreal in 1983. Tessier was originally opposed to having one more society and said that a small travel club would be better. Other voices—particularly Ian Munro—prevailed, and the Society was originally called the International Society of Craniomaxillofacial Surgery, a mistake which was rectified at the Oaxaca meeting, where Hugo Obwegeser was made a full member as he should have at the beginning.

The Founding Members of the Society were Ernesto Caroni, David David, Milton Edgerton, Ian Jackson, Bengt Johansen, Henry Kawamoto, Joe McCarthy, Daniel Marchac, Ian Munro, Joe Murray, Fernando Ortiz-Monasterio, Jorge Psillakis, Ken Salyer, Michel Striker, Paul Tessier, Jacques van de Meulen, Linaton Whitaker, and S. Anthony Wolfe.

The Society is the world's leading body for craniofacial surgery and now has members from over 30 countries worldwide, and its biennial meeting is obligatory for all active craniofacial surgeons.

Dealing with the other interested group - call them oral and maxillofacial surgeons, or Kieferchirugien—still presents some delicate moments, but the situation has been eased somewhat by the requirement that a candidate show documentation of 200 transcranial cases for full membership.

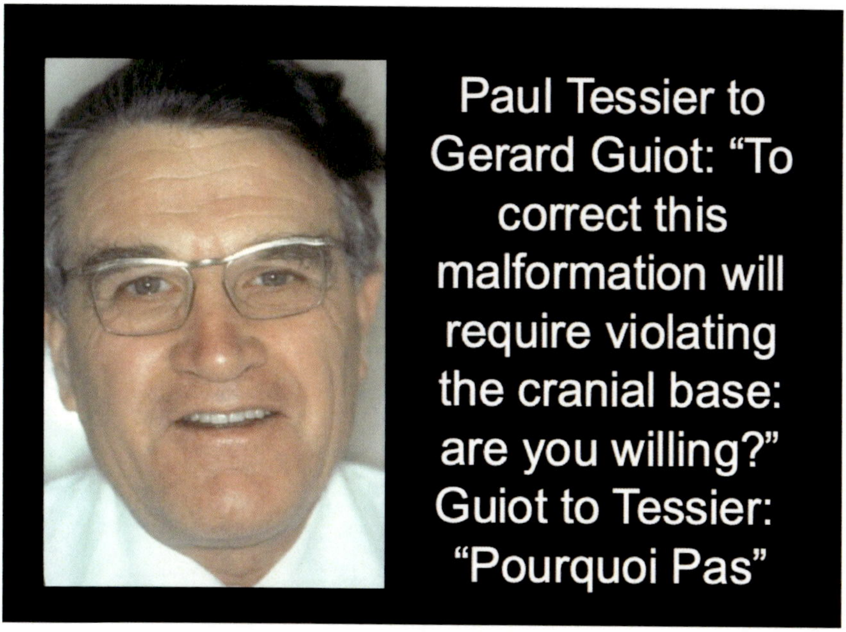
Paul Tessier to
Gerard Guiot: "To
correct this
malformation will
require violating
the cranial base:
are you willing?"
Guiot to Tessier:
"Pourquoi Pas"

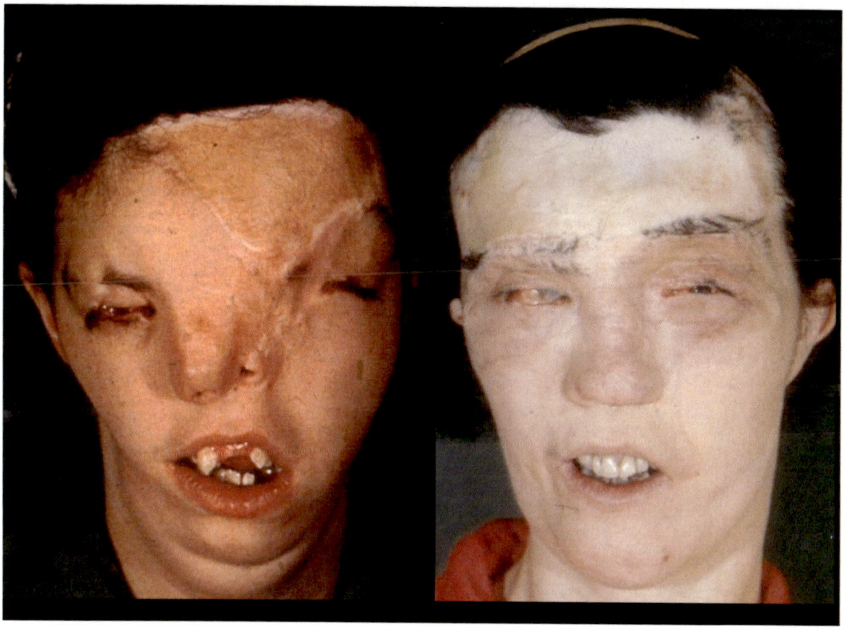

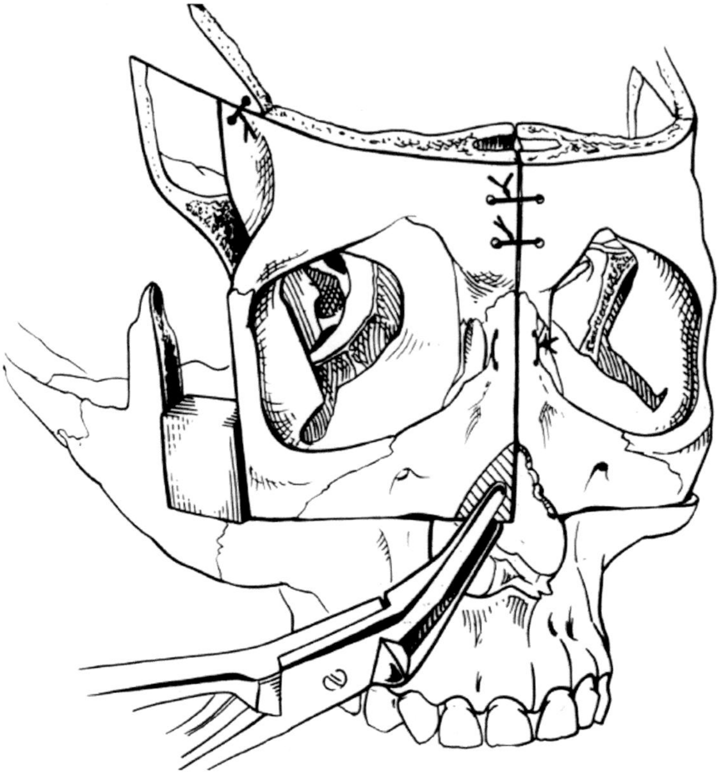

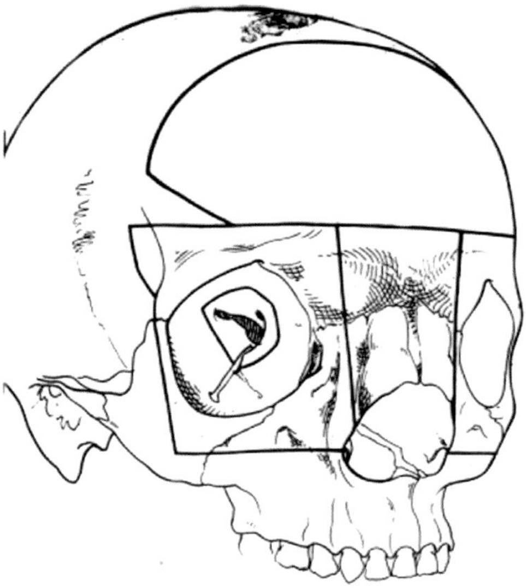

The juries.

Tessier first presented his work at the French Meeting in Monpelier in 1966 but he remained unknown to the English-speaking surgeons. It was not until 1967 at the international meeting in Rome that the enormity of what he had accomplished became evident to the Anglophone community. He was swamped by visitors, so he arranged two teaching sessions which he called "CHOC 1" (1967 and "CHOC II" 1969). CHOC was the acronym for Chirurgie Orbito Cranial, or Orbito Cranial Surgery.

For CHOC 2, the leading surgeons from North America and Europe were invited for a week of live surgery and lectures on the entire field of craniofacial surgery, at the end of which they were asked to vote as a jury on whether or not Tessier should continue.

Return from Paris

In July of 1975 I returned to Miami. I was given a small office in Millard's building and at first spent most of my time helping the residents at Jackson and the VA. There was a lot of facial trauma, so this turned out to be a good proving ground for Tessier's principles.

Quite a few craniofacial cases had been collected for me when I was in Paris, so I started off with a Le Fort 3 in a girl with Pfeiffer syndrome one day and a hypertelorism the next. Larry Page, who I had known when he was a neurosurgical resident at Boston Children's did the neurosurgical part, which for the Le Fort 3 consisted of two burr holes in the temporal fossa to protect the temporal lobes (Tessier's SOS or semi-open skull) and both cases took 12 hours.

For the first few years I did my craniofacial cases at Jackson, but was unhappy with the situation there since I could not get a guaranteed ICU bed and I did not want to send these cases to the floor after a long intracranial procedure.

Miami Children's (Variety Children's then) was growing, and a neurosurgeon named Glenn Morrison joined their staff, and I could have a guaranteed ICU bed. Glenn was a pleasure to work with and I shifted all elective surgery to Children's. I continued to go to Jackson to help the residents with their cases.

One such patient was Emmet ____, who was a medical student in a Caribbean medical school when he was thrown face first from his bicycle into an oncoming bus.

He was airlifted to Jackson and stayed on the oral surgery service for several months before I was consulted. He had a naso orbital ethmoid fracture and his maxilla was floating without any solid connection to his skull.

During that time, he had an intermittent spinal fluid leak which finally stopped. Here I think I made an error in judgement, thinking that an intracranial approach was indicated to seal the dura properly.

The neurosurgeon I was assigned was older and had come to Miami to retire. He insisted on doing the coronal dissection himself, which took 3 hours rather than the usual half hour. He also insisted on having lumber drainage, which I rarely used except if there was an actual CSF leak.

During the case I noticed that the lumbar drain catheter had become dislodged from its drainage bag and was draining directly onto the floor. I did a major procedure with large amounts of iliac and costal bone grafts, fixing the maxilla to the zygomas and the skull, reestablishing the maxillary buttresses with bone grafts, intermaxillary fixation, a large nasal bone graft, and orbital bone grafts.

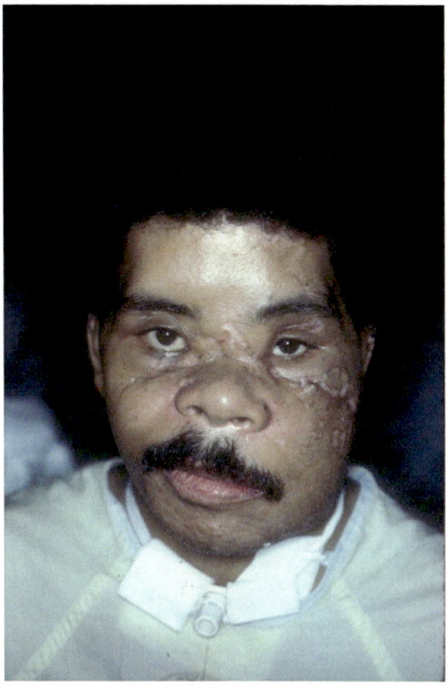
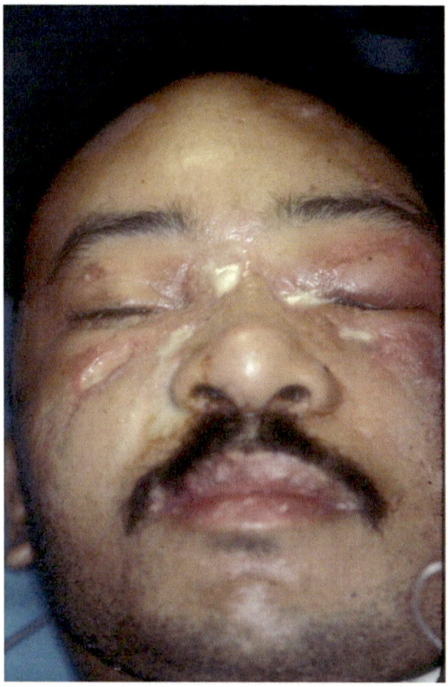
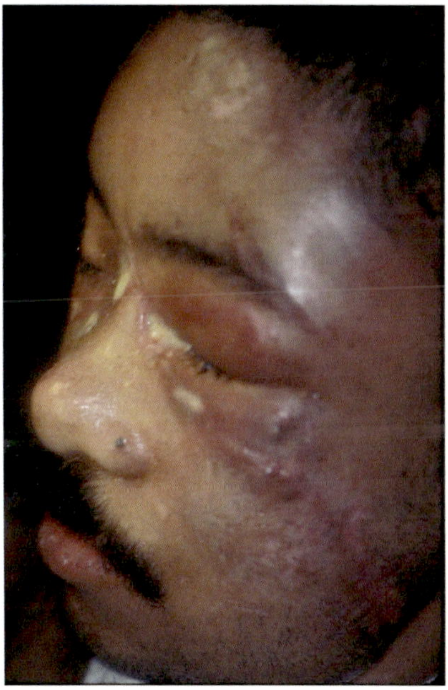
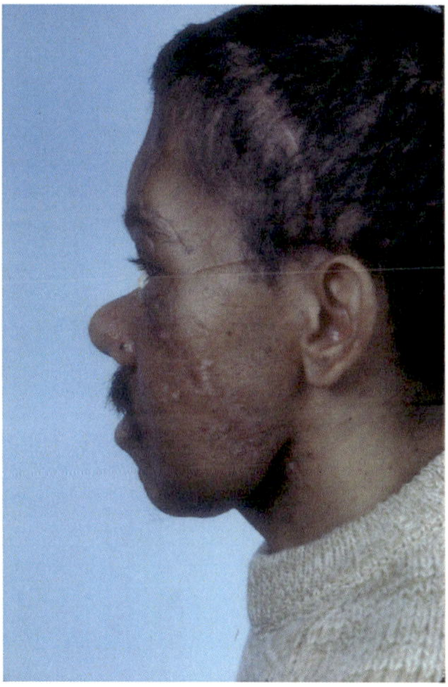

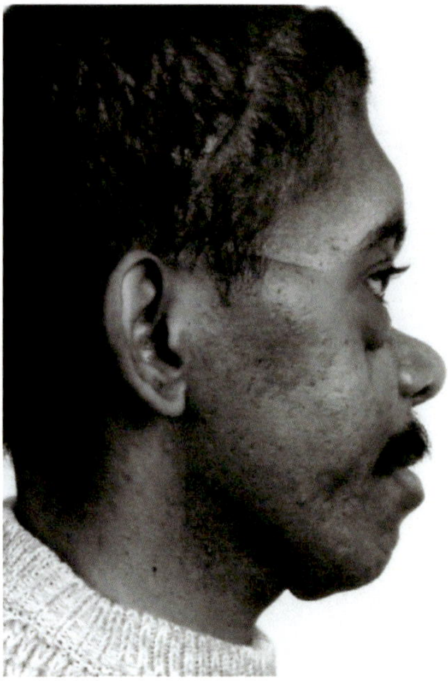

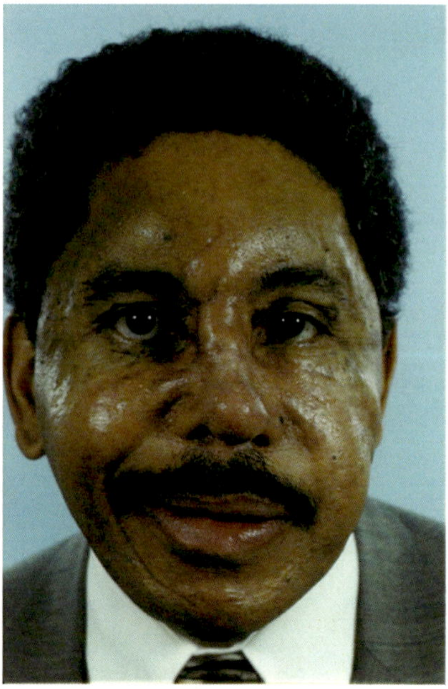

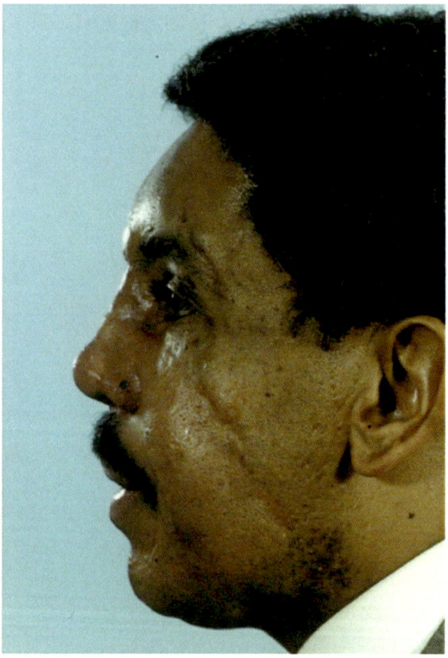

Emmet looked great initially, but at about 3 weeks he became swollen, and there was some drainage from the lower eyelid incisions. When I was out of town the neurosurgeons removed the frontal bone flap - whether this was necessary or not I don't know, since current recommendations are to try to save the flap after a washout with antibiotic solution.

In any event, Emmet was worse that he had been pre-op. I explained to him what lay ahead, and he thanked me, and asked if I knew anyone in Los Angeles who might be able to care for him there since his family were in L.A. I responded there certainly was, and referred him to my friend Henry Kawamoto who finally finished with Emmet after 20 some operations. Emmet is now a practicing orthopedic hand surgeon in L.A. (photos courtesy of Henry Kawamoto MD, DDS).

In retrospect, why did this infection occur? This was in the days before plate and screw rigid fixation. So there may have been some micromovement of the wire osteosyntheses, and then, there is the possibility that the drain catheter exposed to the floor was responsible. In principle what I did was correct, although the craniotomy may not have been needed.

Here is a case of mine, done with Glenn Morrison with rigid plate and screw fixation, but without distraction. For milder cases distraction is not necessary and there is often some distortion of the lateral canthus with distraction.

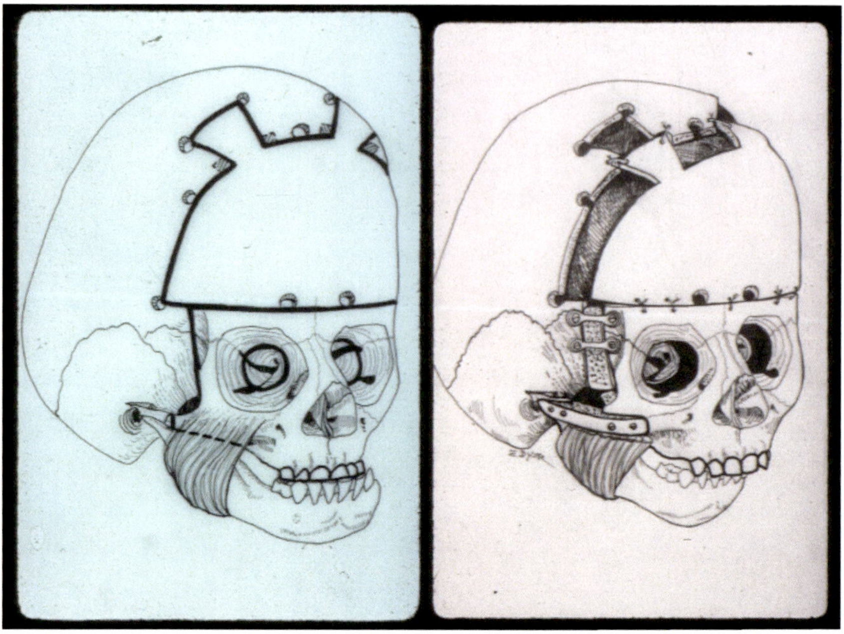

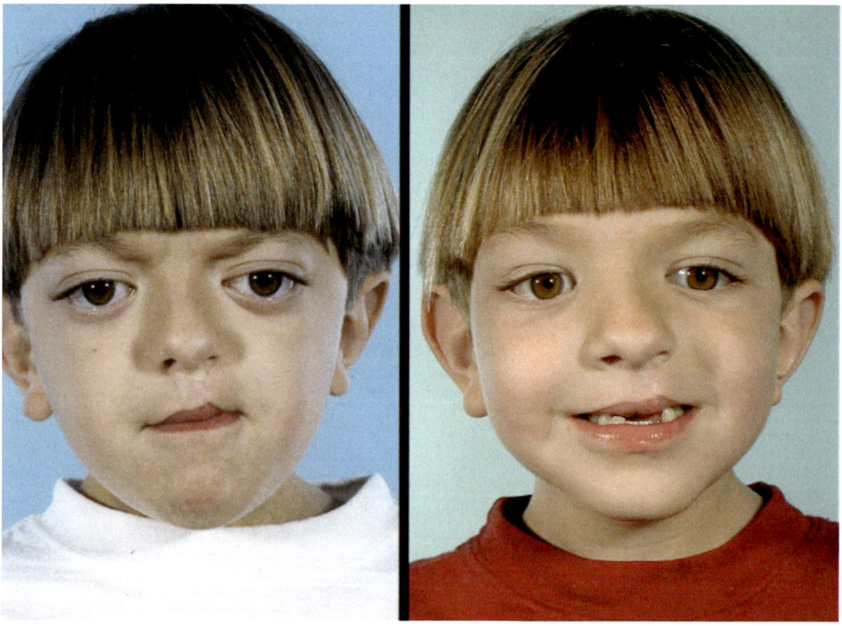

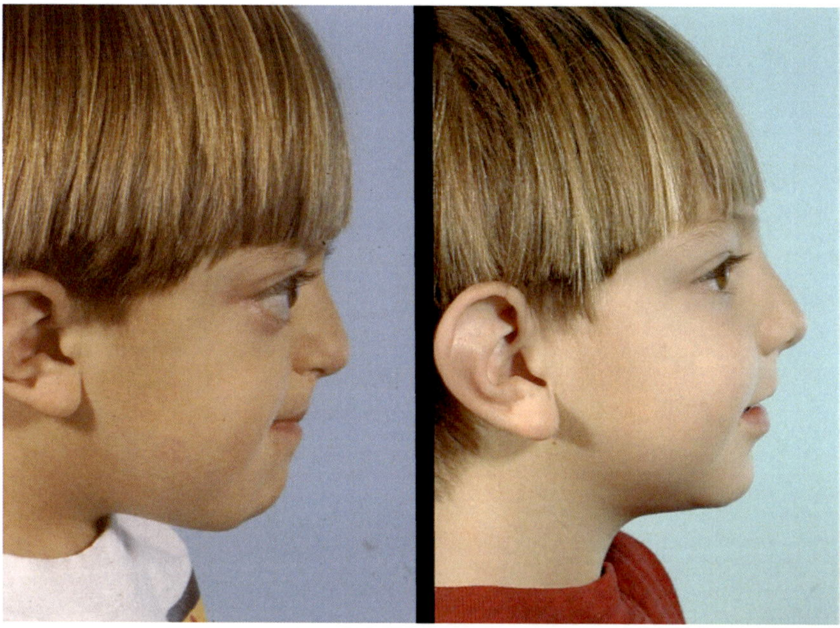

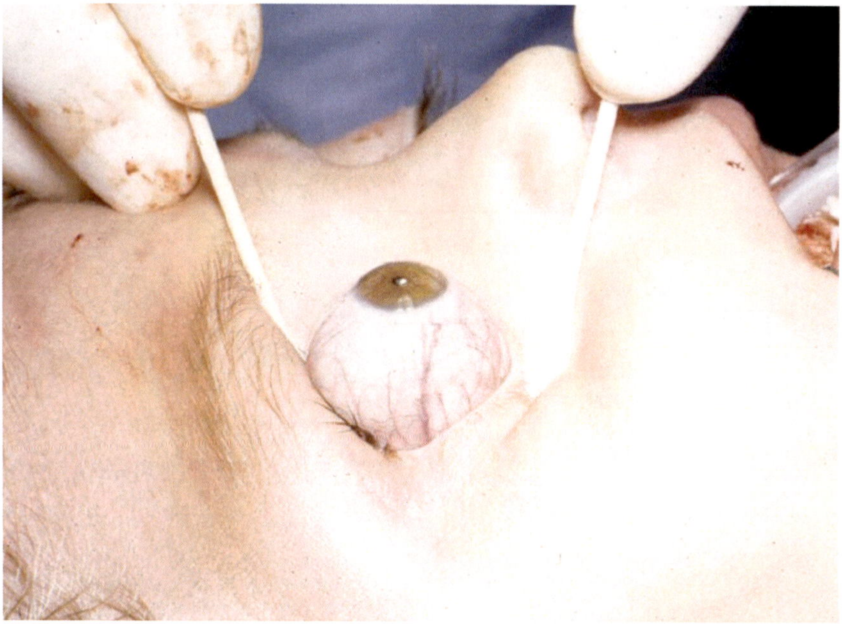

The "Tessier test" demonstrating the degree of proptosis. This cannot be done to a normal individual.

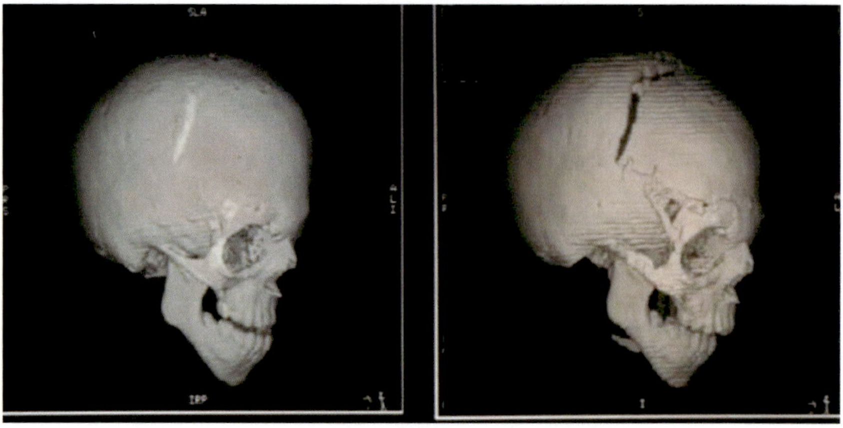

CT scans showing a harmonious advancement with some overcorrection at the alveolar level.

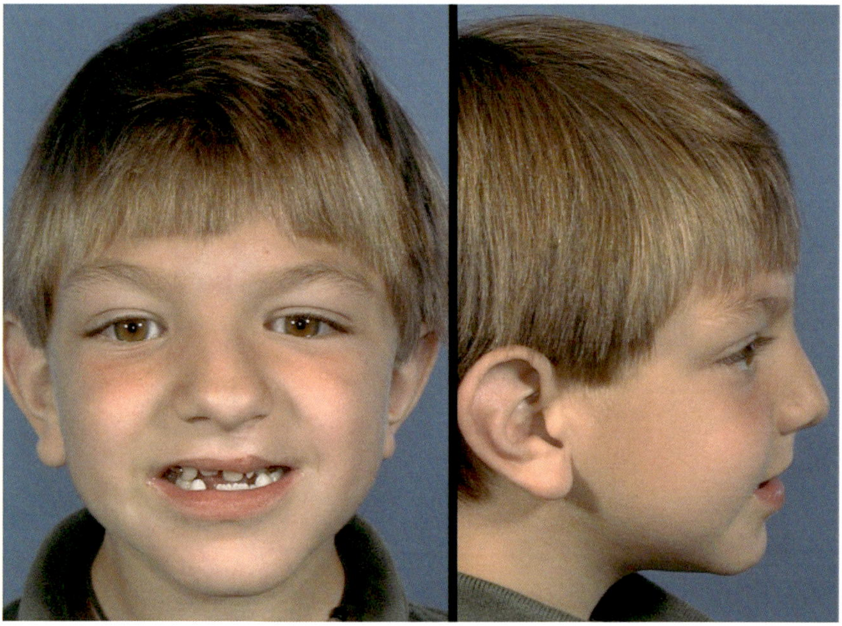

Three-year result and still class 2.

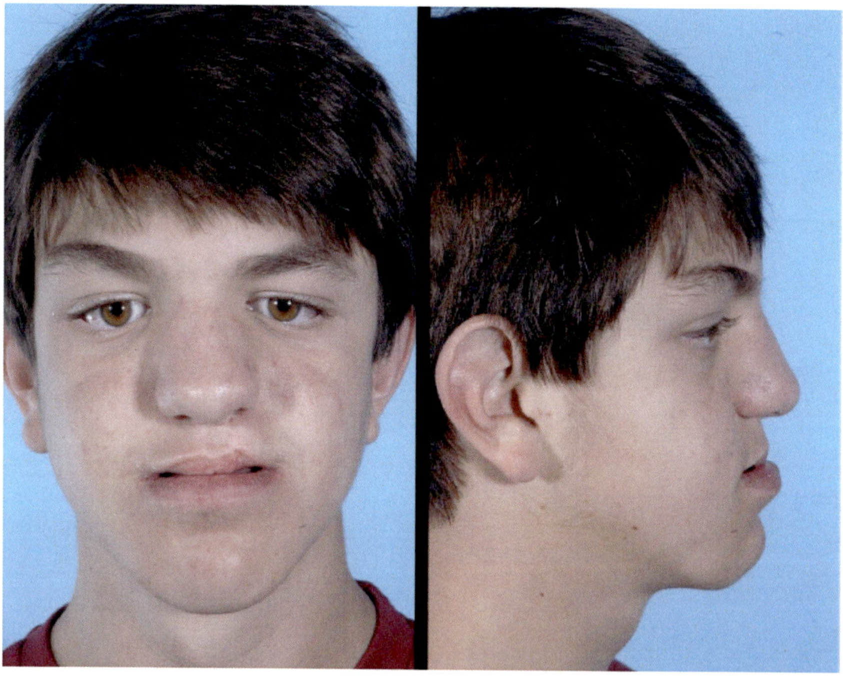

At 10-year result now class 3 due to insufficient maxillary growth.

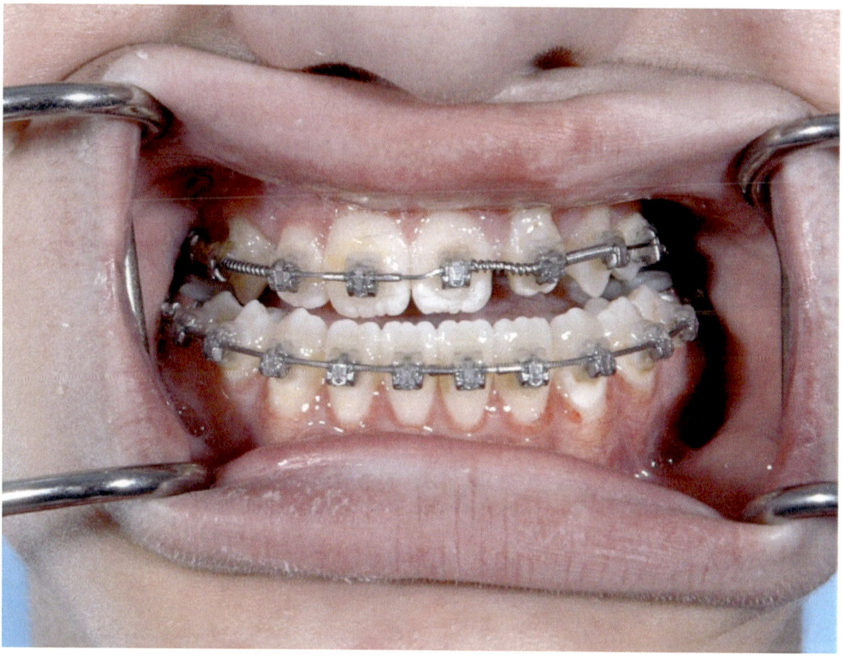

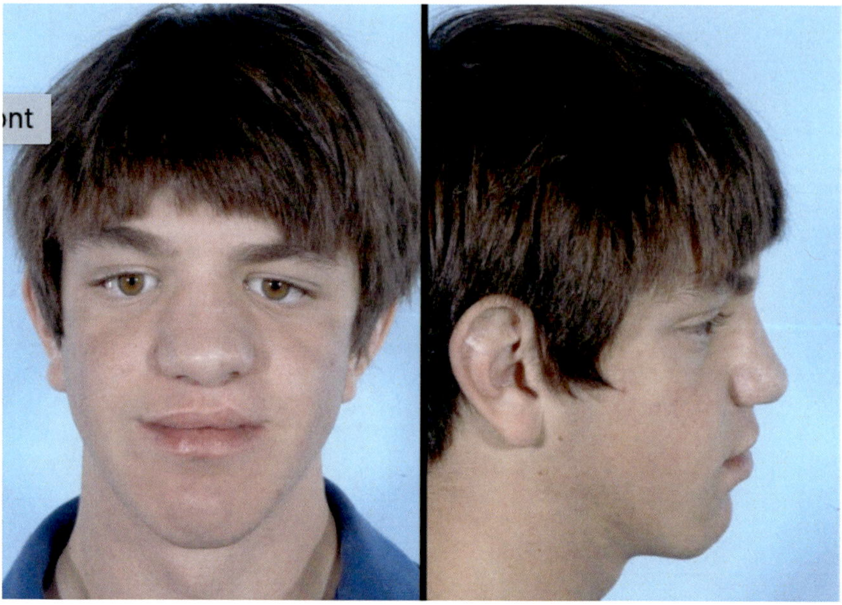

After Le Fort 1 osteotomy in late teens.

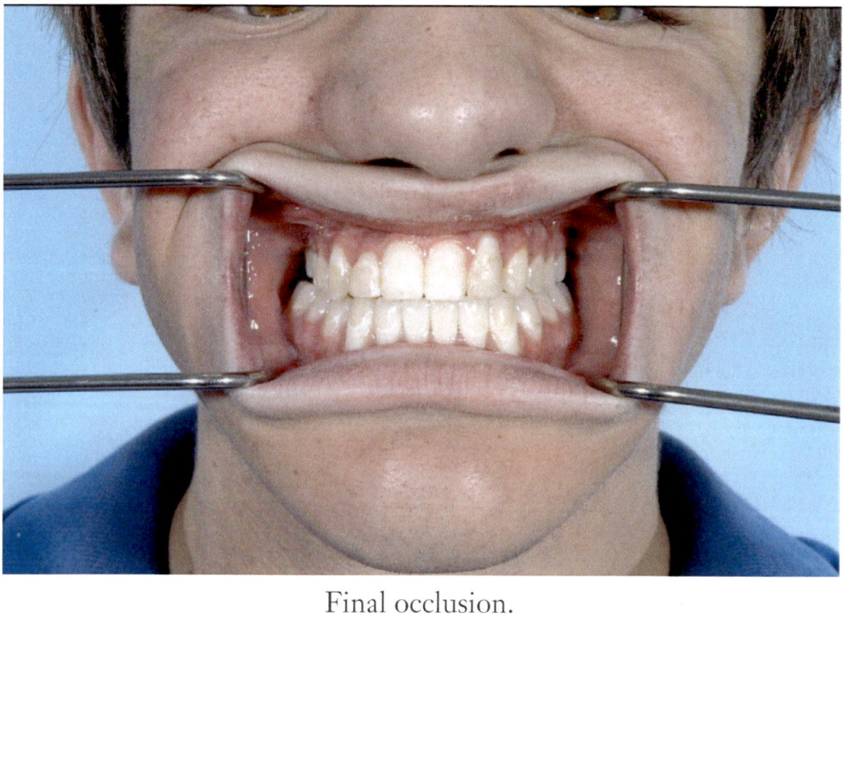

Final occlusion.

During the period of 1980-2000 I continued to do the orthognathic surgery on Dr. Millard's cases, usually a Le Fort 1 maxillary advancement but sometimes a Le Fort 2 or 3, or a two jaw cases involving moving the maxilla forward and the mandible back.

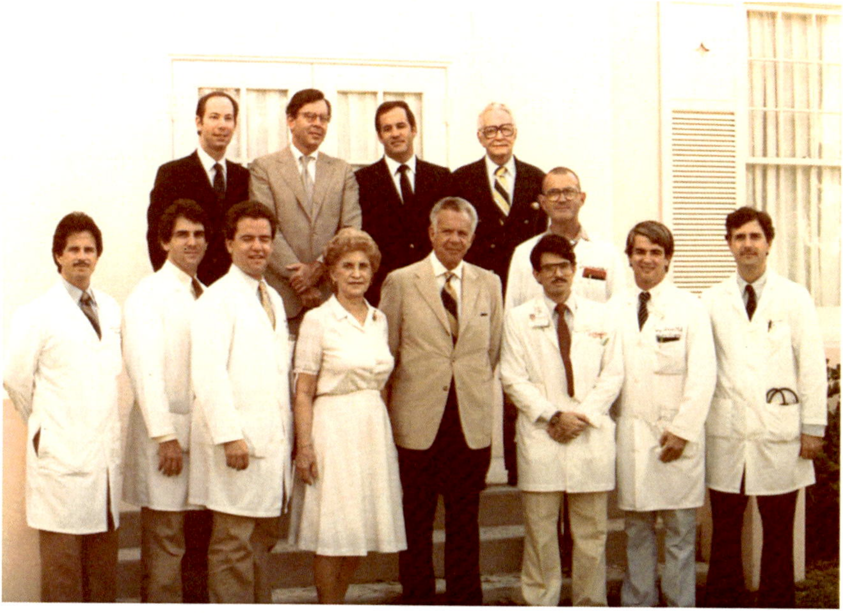

Plastic Surgery staff, Jackson Memorial Hospital, 1980, DRM with Evelyn Shields, second row, Felix Freshwater, SAW, Buster Mullin, John Devine.

During that period if a patient with a cleft lip came to me I would pass the case on to Dr. Millard, since he was after all the world's greatest cleft surgeon, but towards the end of that period I realized that Dr. Millard was nearing retirement and I would have to start doing primary clefts myself. So, I took up primary clefts around 2000, following Dr. Millard's methods as closely as possible. Initially I used the Latham device, a device pinned to the maxilla with a screw which would gradually bring the cleft maxillary segments into close enough abutment that the alveolar cleft could be closed. I did not like the Latham appliance - I needed to put the child asleep to pin the device in place and had to take all of the calls from the parents.

One day in 2001, a young Columbian dentist named Martha Mejia came by the office and asked if I was interested in having her do NAM (naso-alveolar molding), which gradually moved the segments by weekly changes of maxillary splints. She had been working in Dr. Berkowitz's office studying the dental casts of Millard's Latham patients. With Martha's help, we arrived at our current protocol: initiation of NAM at several weeks of age, weekly visits until the alveolar gap is down to 2-3 mm, placing the nasal outrigger at several months, and having the patient ready for surgery at about 6-months, closure of the alveolar cleft and anterior palate with closure of the nasal floor, nasal correction with the McComb technique which consisted of separation of skin from the alar cartilage through the columellar base and alar base, piercing the alar cartilage about 3 mm lateral to the columella through the vestibule with a suture mounted on a Keith needle brought through the skin at the contralateral nasion and the cartilage locked in its new position with several vestibular effacement sutures begun intranasally, passing through the alar crease, then back through the same needle hole to be tied intranasally. And then nostril stents for a week.

After I had been doing primary clefts for a year or two, I sent some of my results to Dr. Millard for his comments. In his response he gave me a good grade for the unilaterals, but not the bilaterals - because I, like "that guy" in Boston (John Mulliken) hadn't used one of his pet operations, the forked flap, to lengthen the columella.

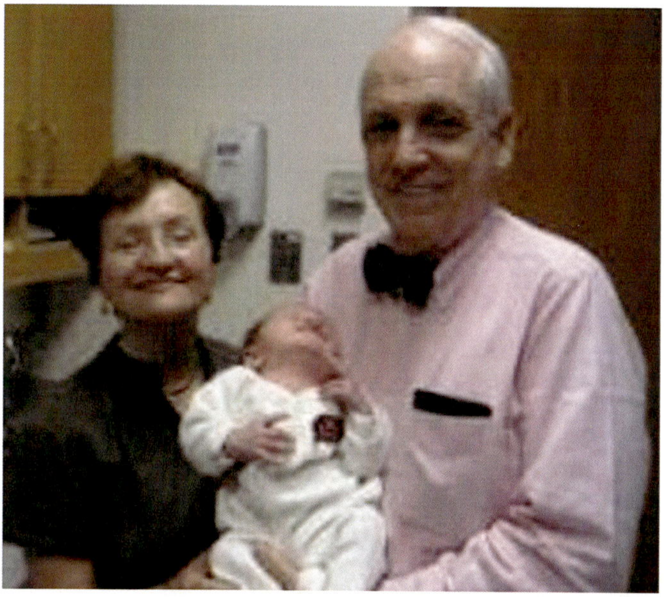

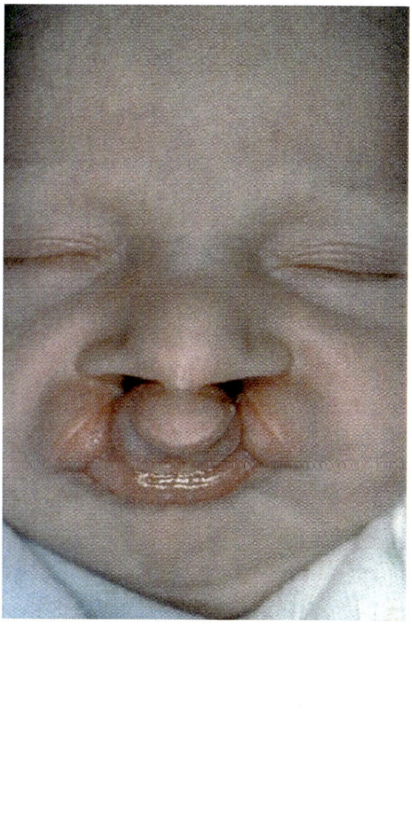

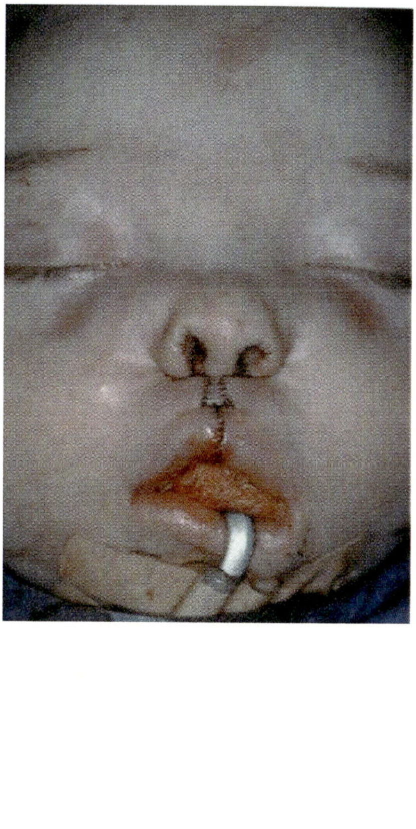

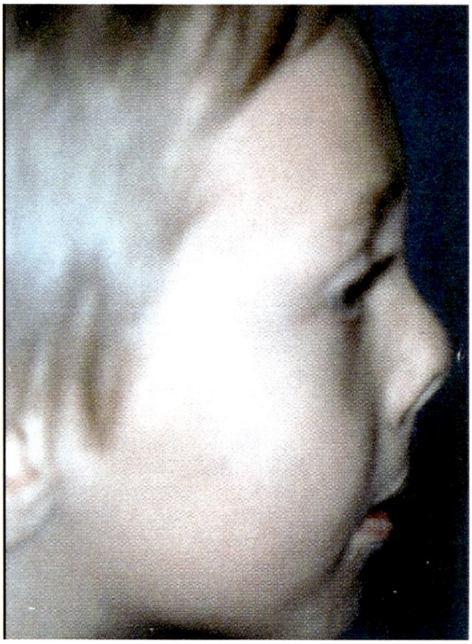

Published case of John Mulliken with normal prolabium ending up a tiny one.

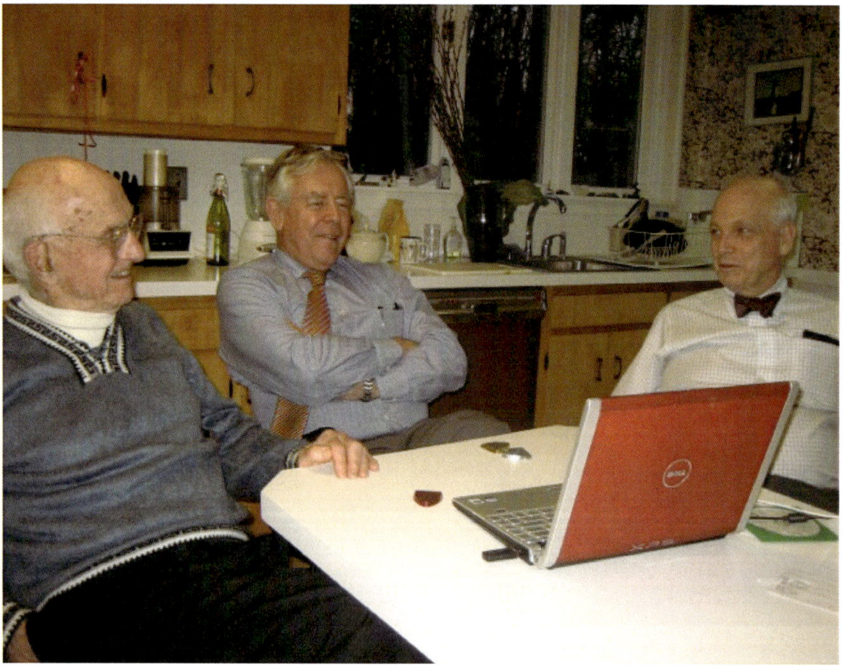

With John Mulliken in Joe Murray's kitchen.

It shows that Millard felt the nasal deformity was due to inadequate skin, when in fact it is the cartilage which was responsible.

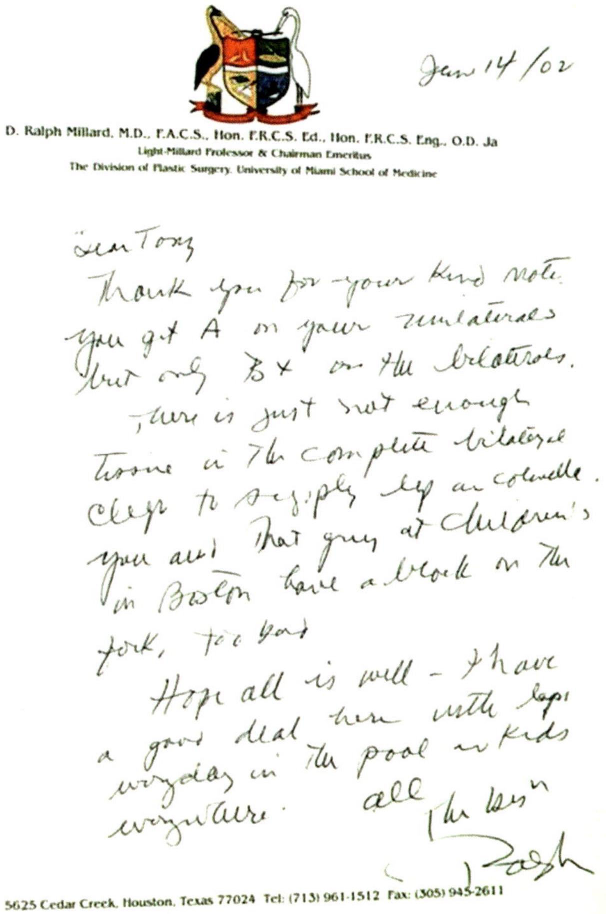

Jan 14/02

D. Ralph Millard, M.D., F.A.C.S., Hon. F.R.C.S. Ed., Hon. F.R.C.S. Eng., O.D. Ja
Light-Millard Professor & Chairman Emeritus
The Division of Plastic Surgery, University of Miami School of Medicine

Dear Tony
Thank you for your kind note.
You got A on your unilaterals
but only B+ on the bilaterals.
There is just not enough
tissue in the complete bilateral
cleft to supply lip an columella.
You and that guy at Children's
in Boston have a block on the
fork, too bad
Hope all is well - I have
a good deal here with laps
everyday in the pool w kids
everywhere. all the best
Ralph

5625 Cedar Creek, Houston, Texas 77024 Tel: (713) 961-1512 Fax: (305) 945-2611

In the bilateral cases I sent him, the columella was normal with bilateral McComb procedures, but the lobule, the point of maximal tip projection, was inadequate.

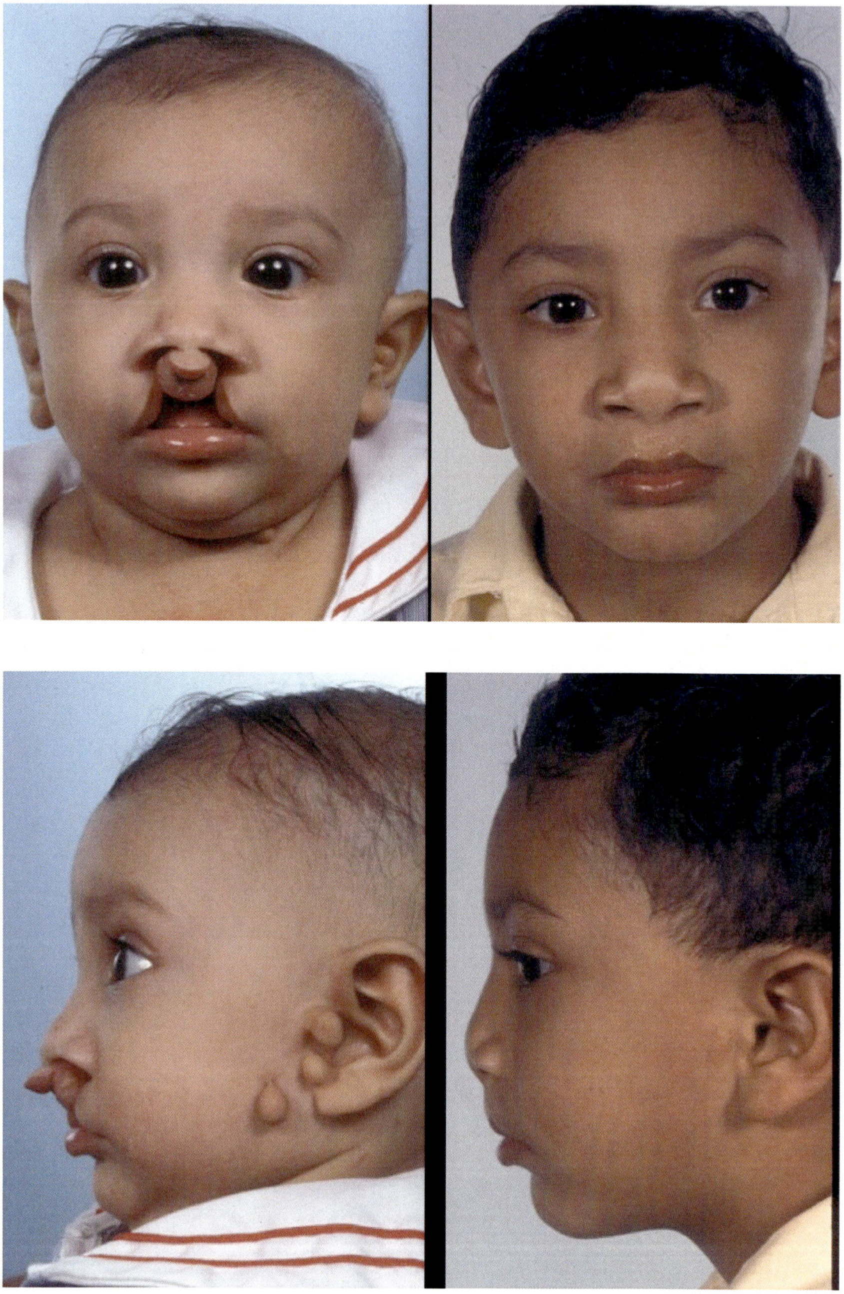

One stage repair done by Millard with forked flap lengthening of columella. I did a minor revision of the nose. There is a masterful artificial Cupid's bow, but the lip is tight and lacks a pout.

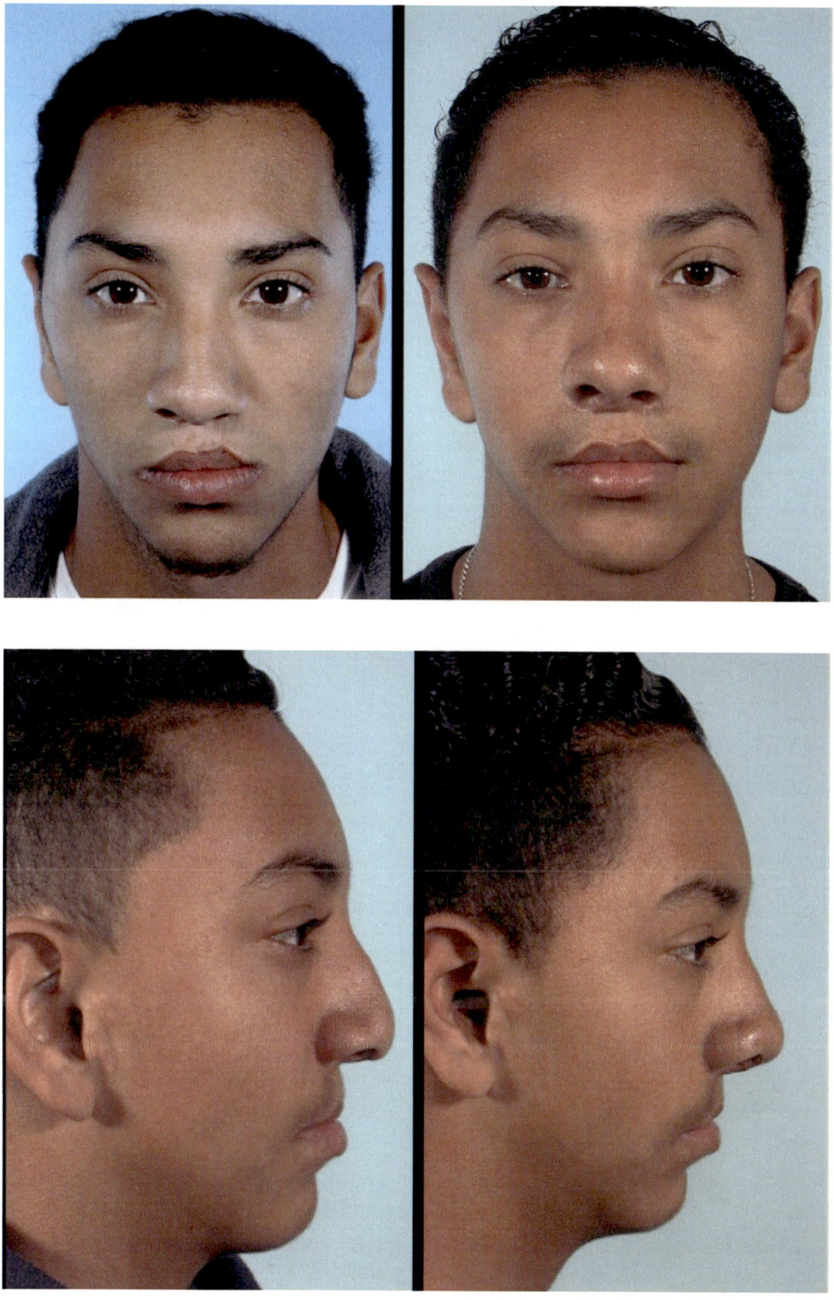

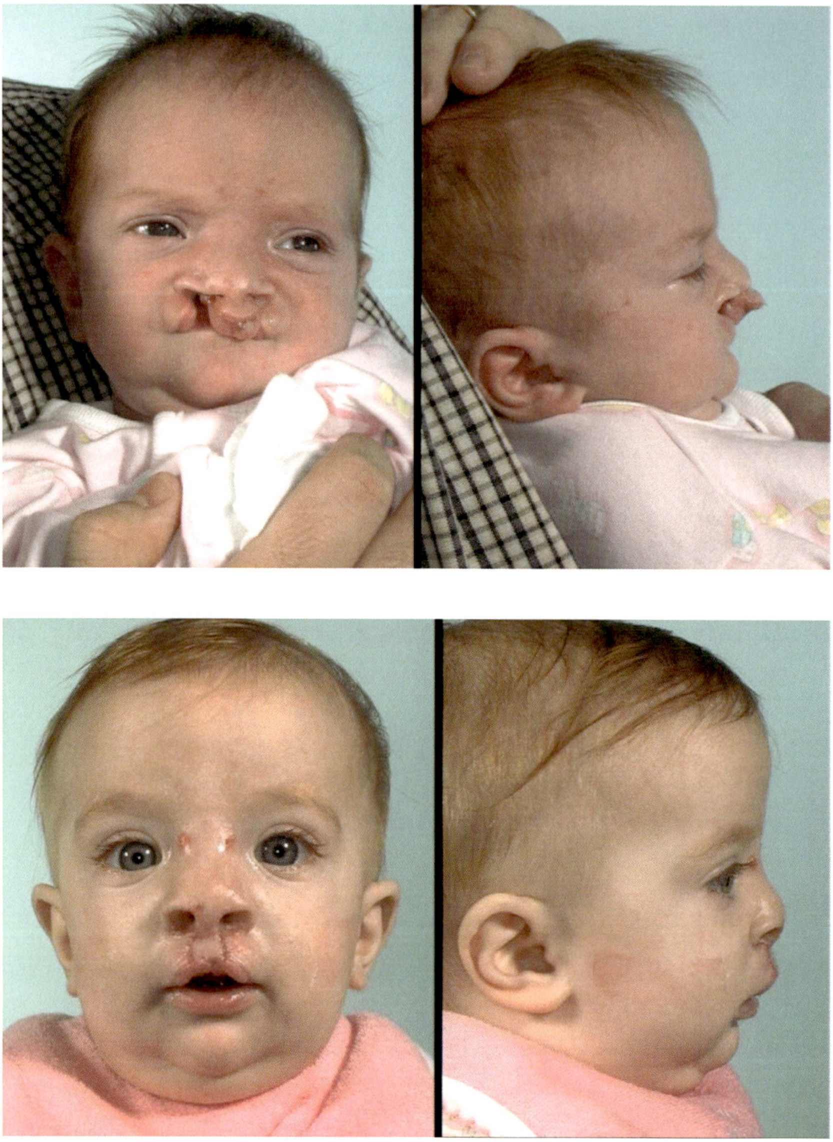

One stage repair done by me. The prolabium is boxy and the lobule deficient.

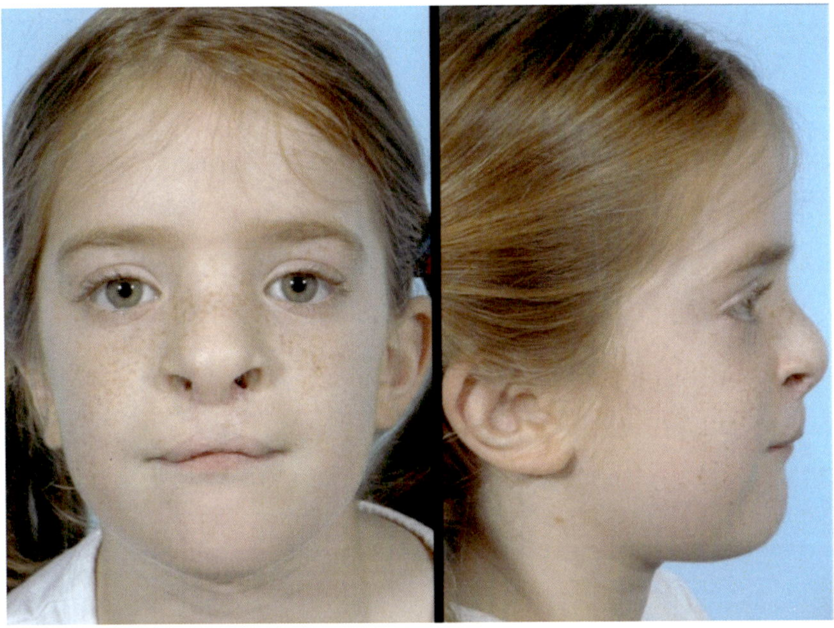

None of these cases, not Mulliken's, not Millard's and certainly not mine do I consider to be a good result. The upper lips are short and tight, and the premaxilla ventroflexed. The columellas are not normal, and the lobules are deficient.

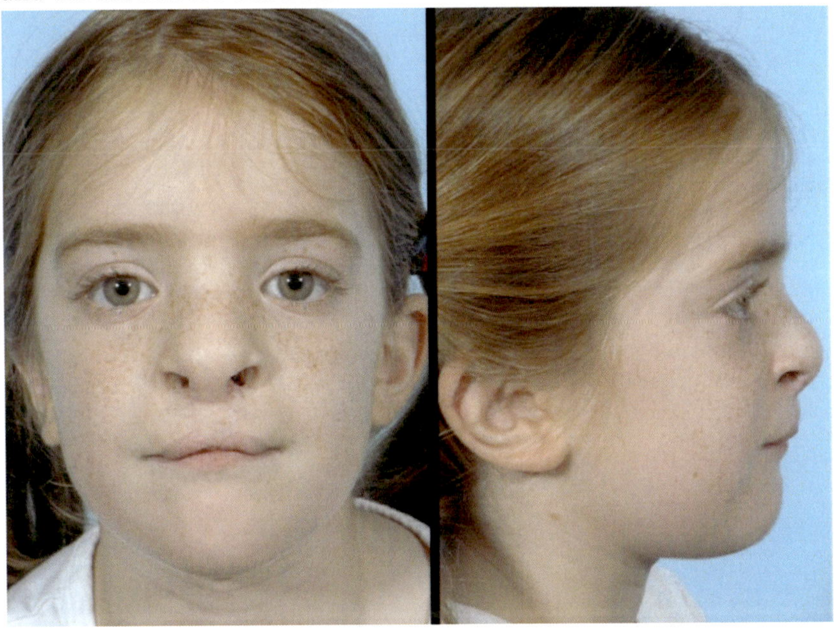

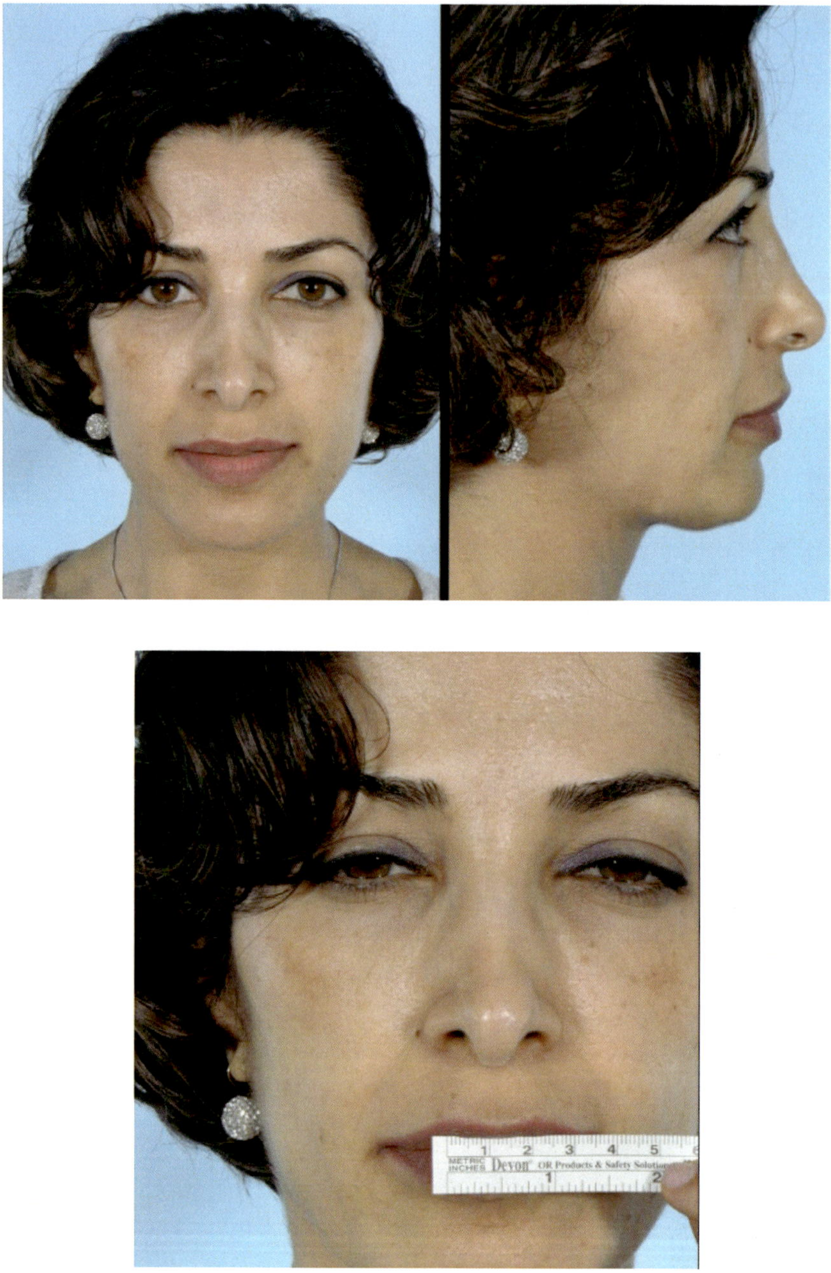
METRIC
INCHES
Devon

A new approach for complete bilaterals.

The results for the unilaterals were routinely good using Millard's rotation advancement with minor modifications. I did not incise around the alar base as far as he did and used the c-flap to create a medial foot plate rather than place it into the columella. And, as mentioned, I used the McComb method rather than Millard's direct suture through a vestibular incision.

The problem was with the complete bilaterals: none of the results with a one-stage repair were good, not mine, not Millard's, not Mulliken's. The reasons were multiple:

1. The primary defect that needs correction in a cleft lip is lengthening of the lip on the cleft side. A rotation advancement does that and places the scar in symmetry with the normal philtra column.
2. A one stage repair leaves the lip short on both sides, and instead of a curved, shield shaped philtrum, provides a short, rectangular one.
3. The native white roll is lost, an artificial cupid's bow is created.
4. The orbicularis muscle is sutured together beneath the prolabium, often under tension.
5. The lateral lip elements (except in the Manchester where prolabial vermillion is not dissected away) are brought together in an attempt to create a tubercle.
6. In addition John Mulliken, using Leslie Farkas' anthropometric date, advised trimming the prolabium to a length of 4.5 mm, discarding large portions of the prolabium.

I arrived at our current protocol incrementally. There were many cases of asymmetric bilaterals, with a complete cleft on one side and an incomplete on the other. It did not make sense to do these cases with a one-stage repair, as advocated by John Mulliken. I began doing the complete side first just as if it were a unilateral cleft, then three months later closed the incomplete side. The results were excellent.

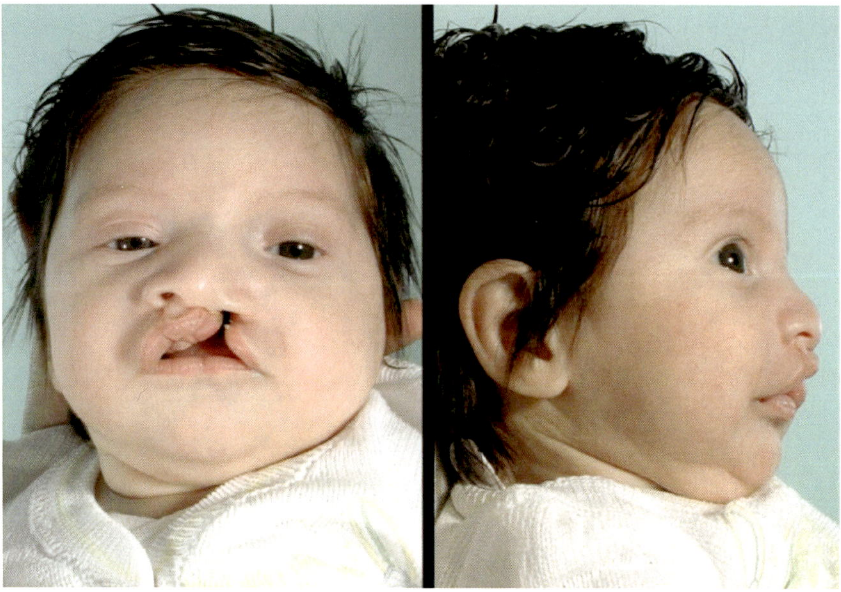

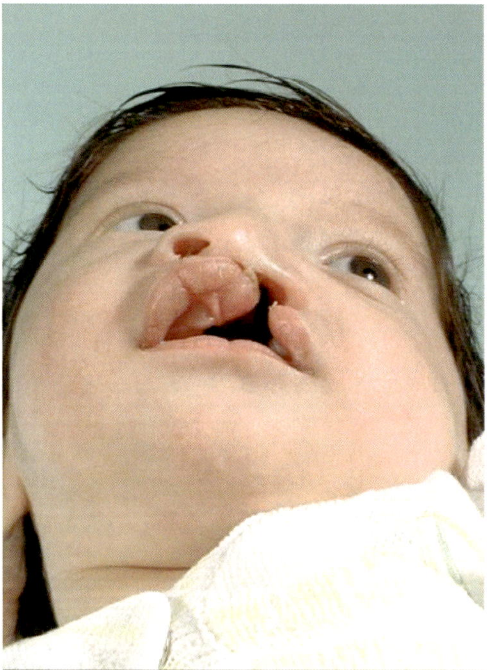

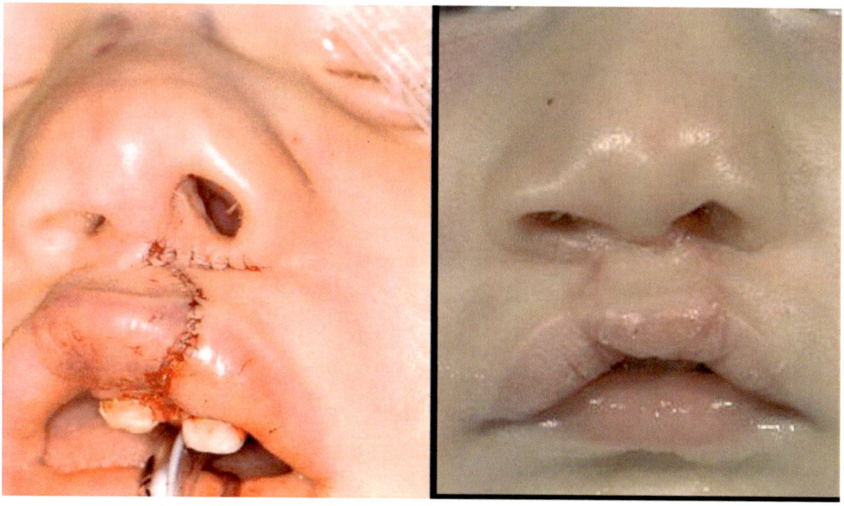

After closure of complete cleft first.

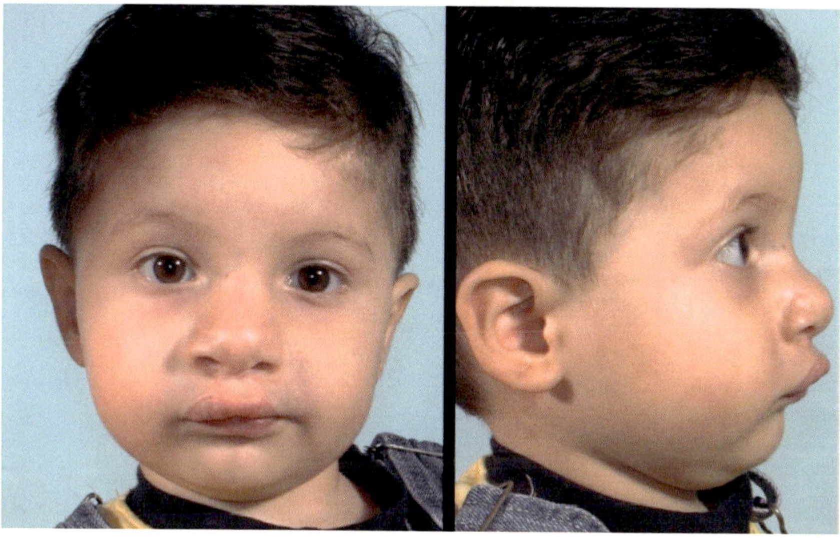

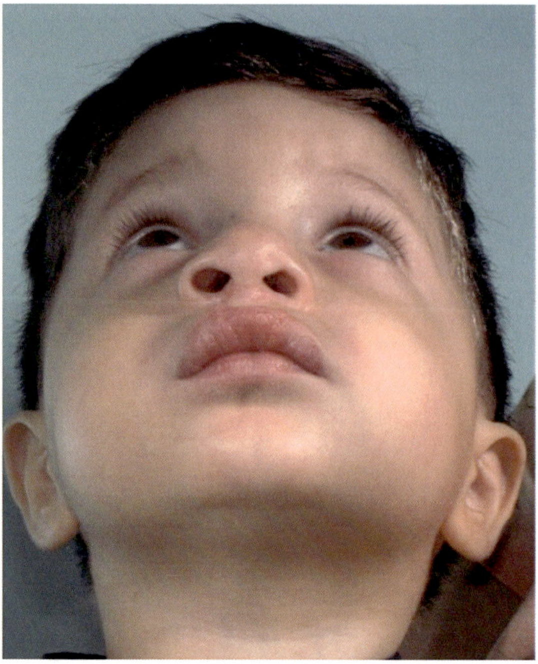

After closure of lesser cleft on right. The lip is full and pouting, and the nose normal. Symmetry is not difficult to obtain.

Finally, I got the nerve to do a complete bilateral in stages. After I finished the second side, I was struck with the fact that not only had I lengthened the lip, but the nose was normal—both in terms of the columella, but also with a normal lobule.

Not immodestly, this was the best result I had ever seen in a complete bilateral cleft: there was a normal nose, including the iobule and columella, a lengthened lip with a normal philtrum, wider than Mulliken's suggested width, but at the upper limits of normal, a pouting lip, well in front of the lower lip on profile, a normal nasolabial angle. I know it is considered poor form to applaud one's own results, and I admit to being guilty.

I applied this method to all complete bilaterals that came to us, and the results were similar.

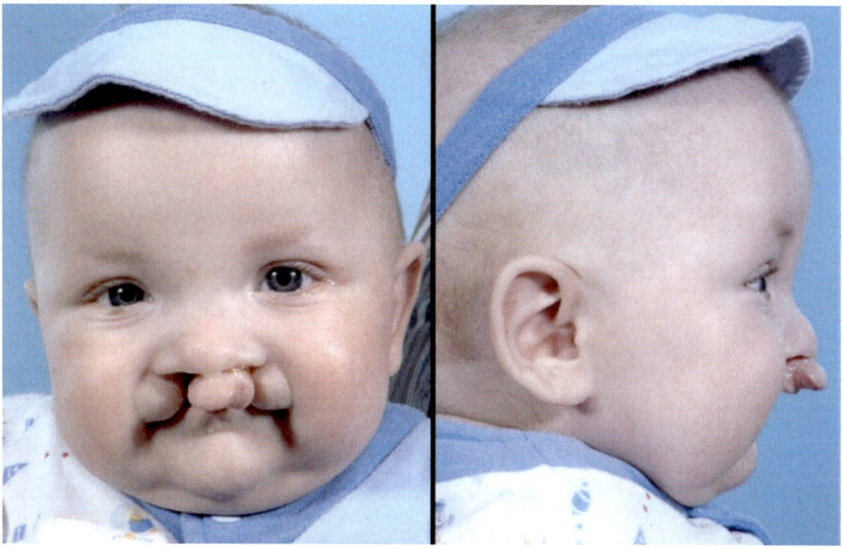

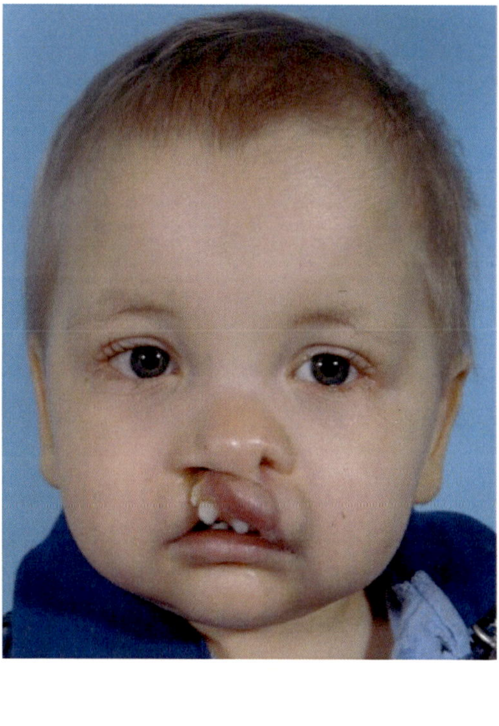

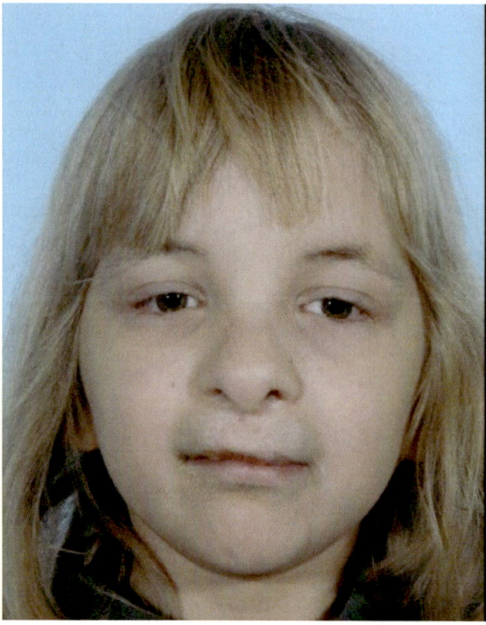

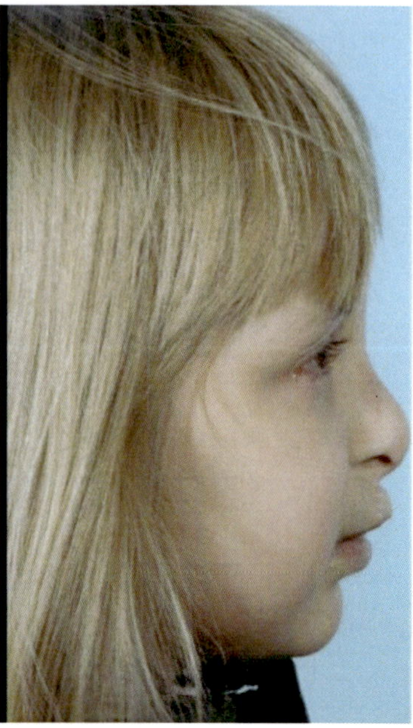

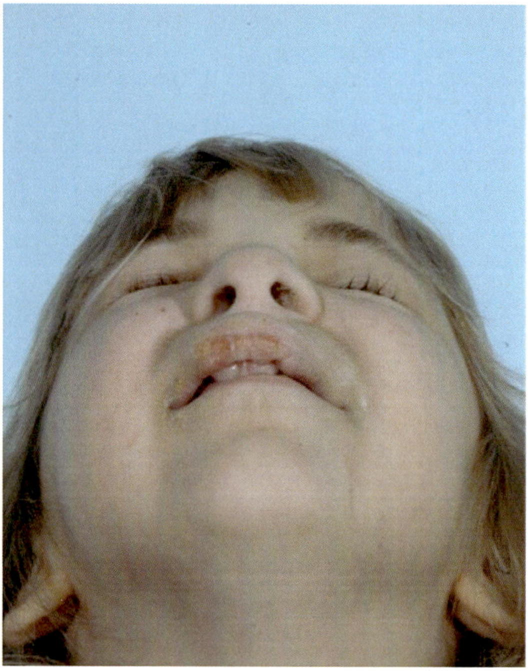

Here is our current protocol:

See patient in neonatal period. Start alveolar moulding at about two weeks. Bring alveolar segments to 2-3 mm gap.

At 3 months begin nasal molding and have patient ready for lip repair at 6 months, with premaxilla in good position. Close wider side with rotation advancement (you can make prolabium any size you want—I prefer wider since less tissue discarded). Gingivoperiosteoplasty (supraperiosteal over tooth roots) with closure of alveolar cleft and anterior palate.

Nasal correction with McComb technique. In short, the same rotation advancement used for a unilateral cleft. The procedure is repeated for the other side after 3 months. The remainder of the palate is closed at 18 months.

There is no expectation that the GPP will result in enough bone formation for orthodontic needs. At 5 years, percutaneous iliac bone grafts are placed into the alveolar gaps - often there is some new bone formation, but not enough.

In a certain percentage of cases, there will be no need for further surgery.

The one minor problem that has been encountered is that in 10-15 percent of cases there will be inadequate bulk to the prolabial vermillion - because there is no muscle in the prolabium of the complete bilateral cleft. A small retroauricular dermofascial graft in these cases can be placed at time of the palate closure or bone graft and that usually corrects the deformity. In one case, there was still a deficiency which was corrected by a mucosal only Abbe flap.

I have been asked about muscle function with this approach since we are suturing the lateral orbicularis muscle to mesoderm. Videos show that there is a good ability to whistle, electromyography would be needed to further delineate the presence of activity. Suturing the lateral orbicularis muscle together beneath the small prolabium is recommended in one-stage repairs, and if done with tension may limit maxillary growth. Boston Children's reports a 76% incidence of Le Fort

1 in their skeletally mature complete bilaterals. We reported on 15 unilaterals and 15 complete bilaterals treated according to our protocol in deciduous dentition, and all were Class 1. This in itself is good reason to switch to staged repairs.

I have wondered what Dr. Millard would say about this approach, since he was so wed to his one stage repair and forked flap for the columellar shortness. I think initially he would pooh pooh the approach, saying that he had done this in the past, but I think that realizing it was his rotation-advancement repeated that would make it easier to accept. He would then without any fanfare adopt the method himself and maybe improve it. Results count.

Finally, why were the noses normal in the staged repairs and abnormal in the one-stage cases? I concluded that when you hike up the alar cartilages at the same time, by McComb technique or whatever, the two crura are fighting for the same space and do not get the same elevation as a single side.

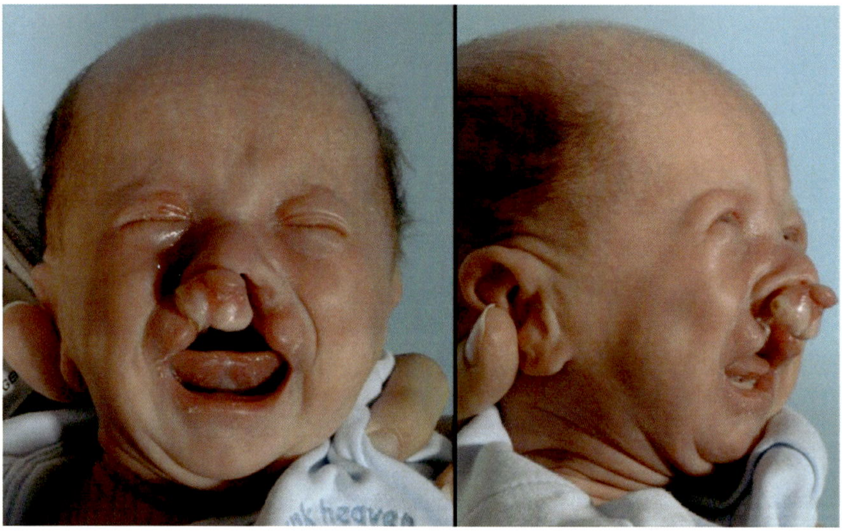

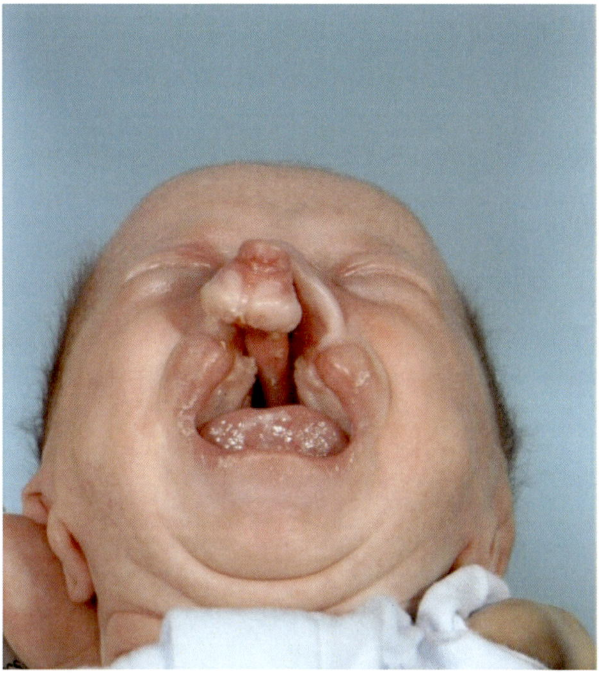

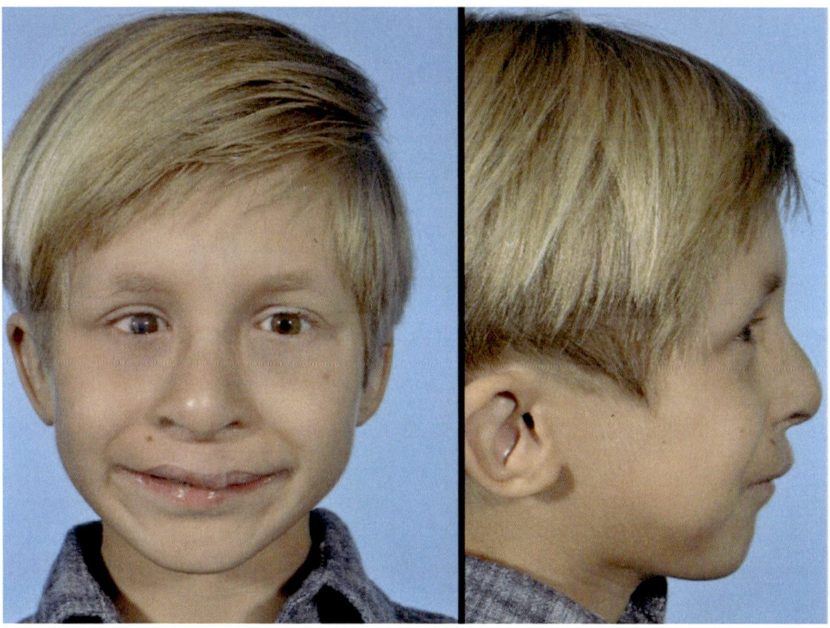

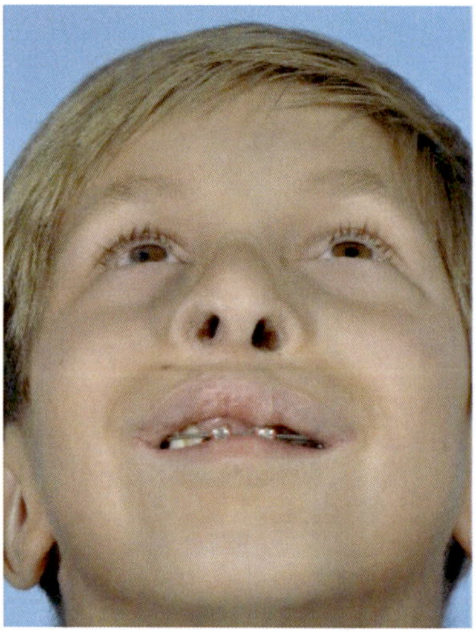

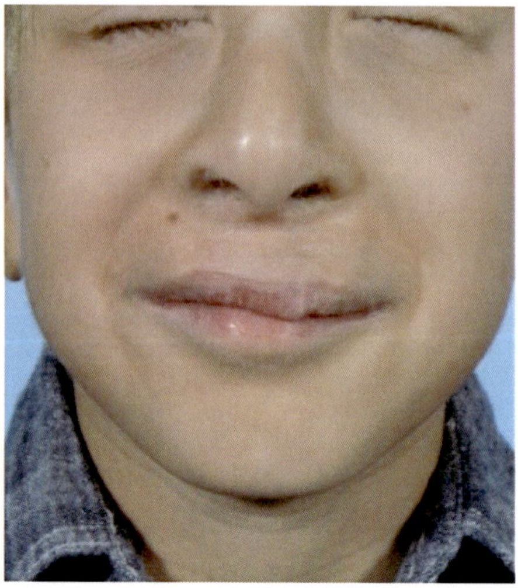

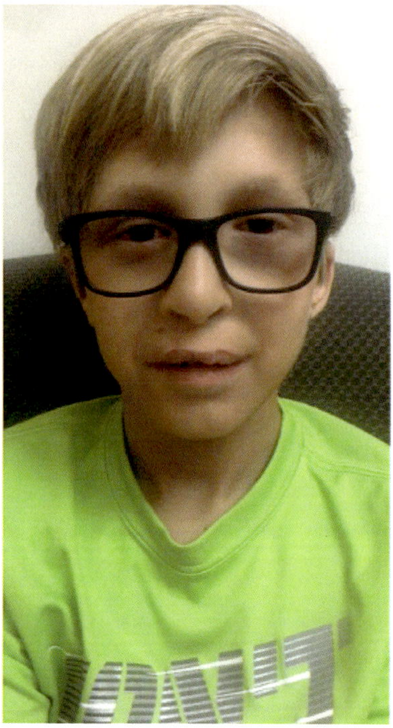

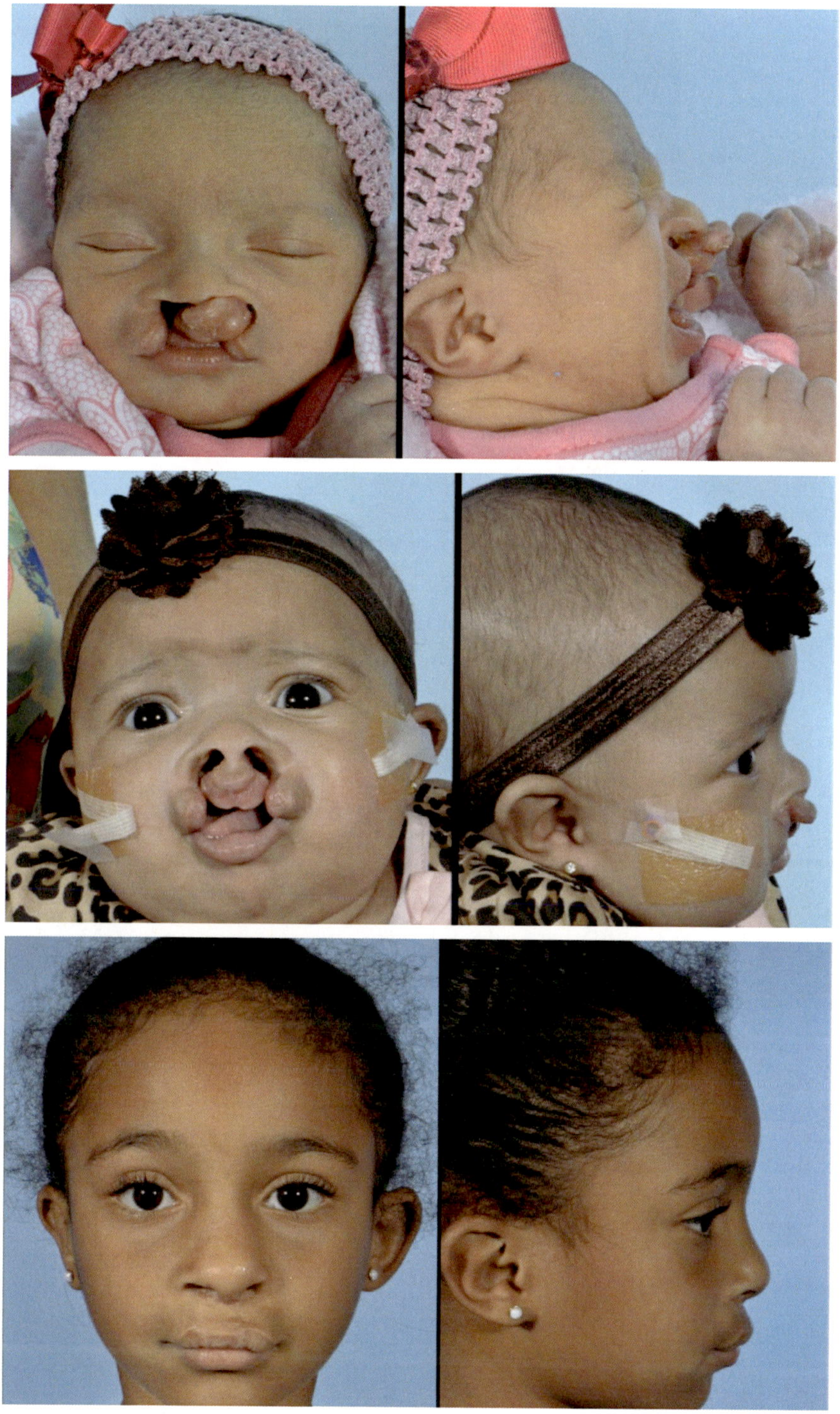

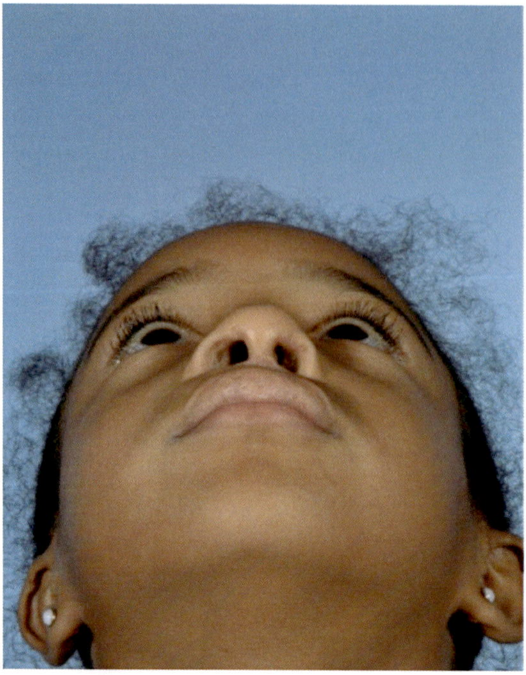

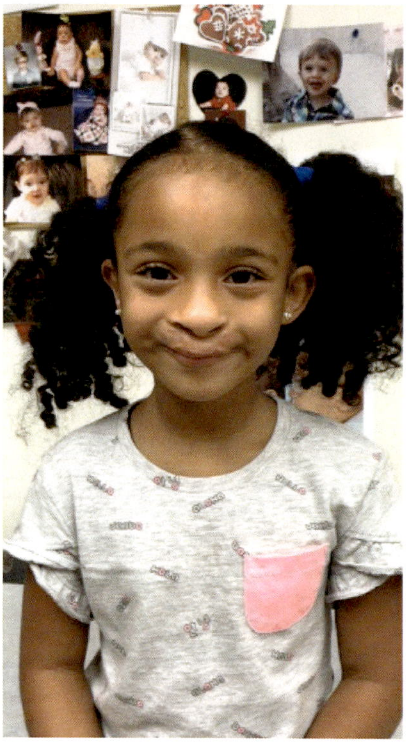

A selection of craniofacial cases are shown, which would not be possible without the teachings of Dr. Millard and Dr. Tessier.

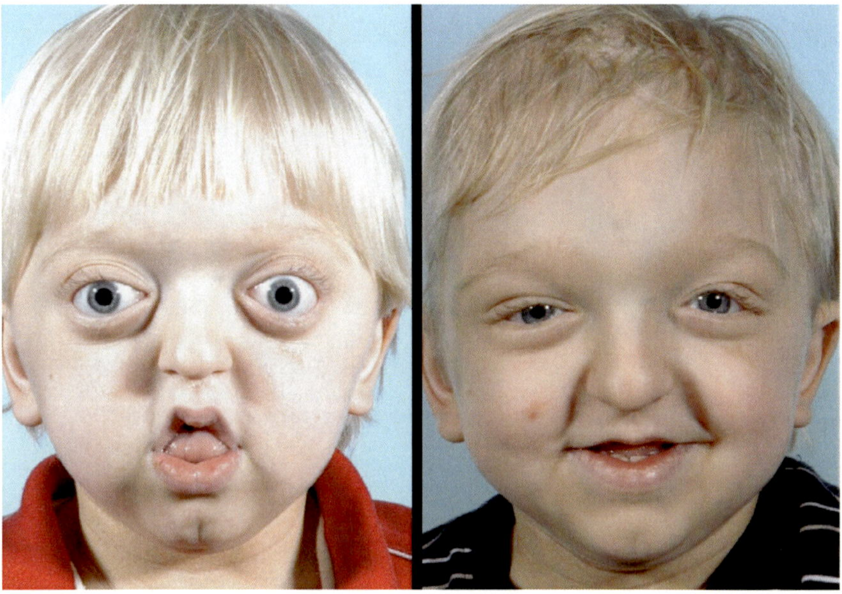

Monobloc frontofacial advancement without distraction at age 5 shown at two weeks post-op.

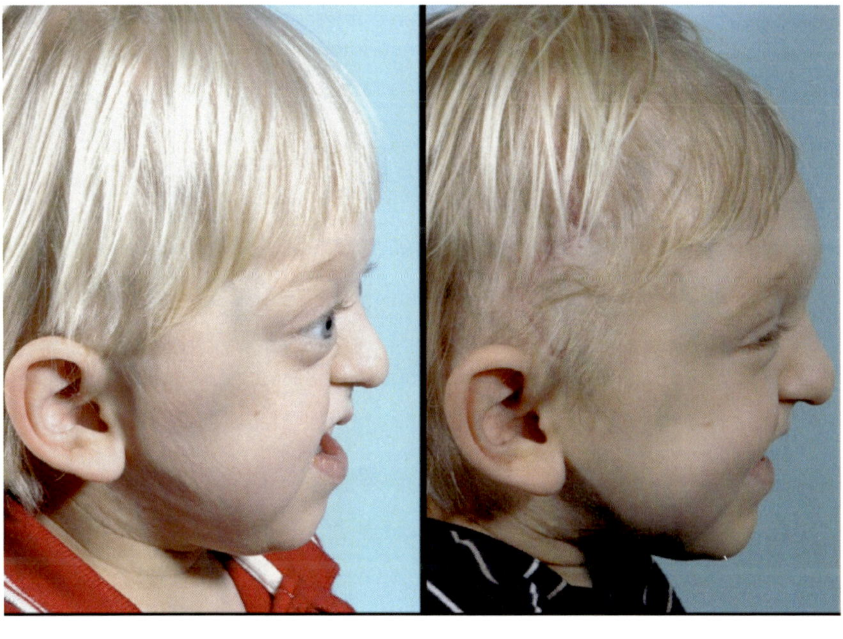

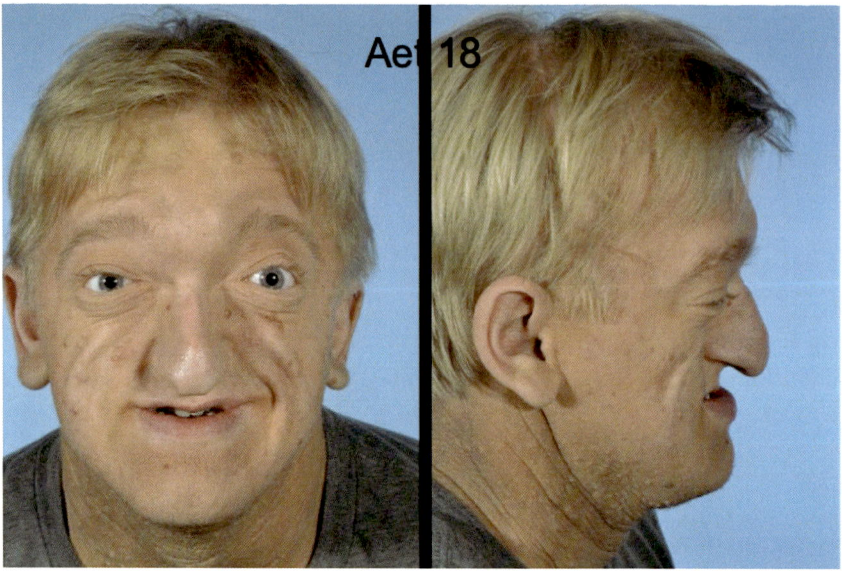

Fronto-orbital correction remains at age 18, but there has been minimal maxillary growth with a resultant severe class 3 deformity.

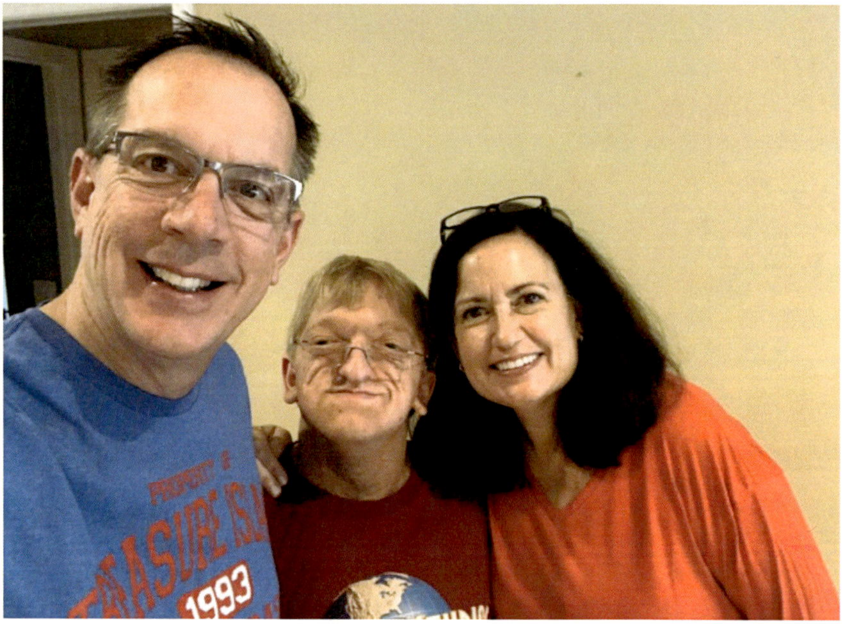

At age 18 the patient could be mistaken for a grandparent of his own parents.

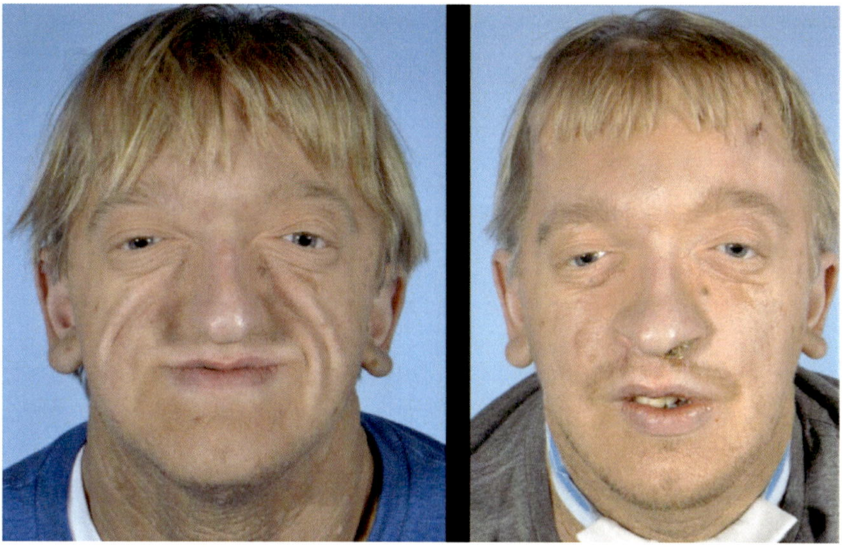

Shown after modified Le Fort 3 advancement which has provided an "internal facelift."

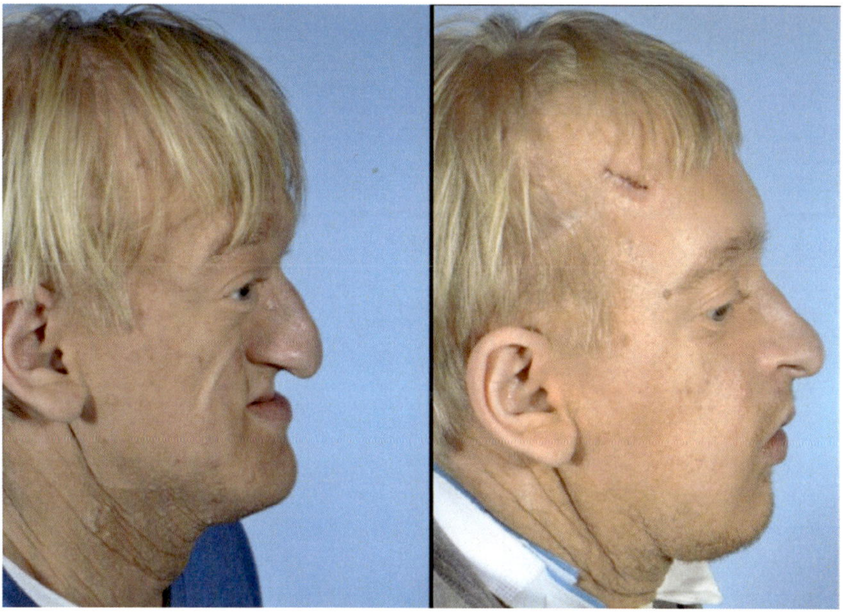

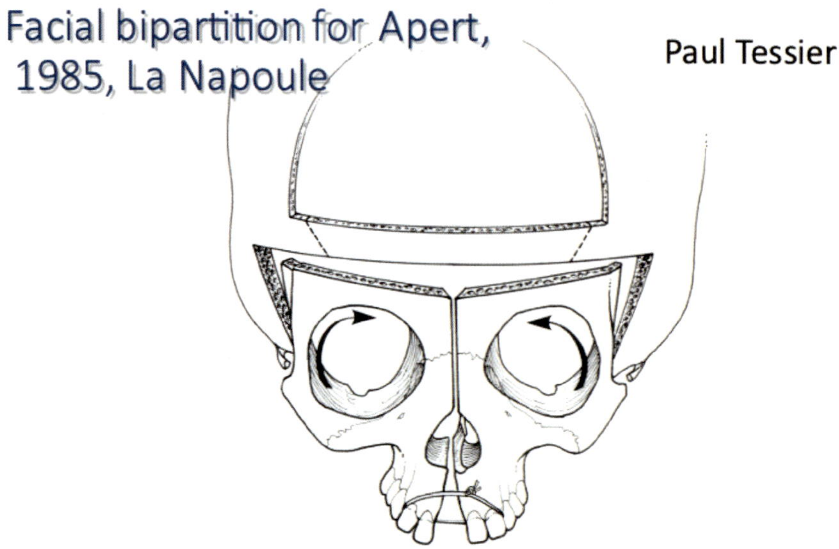

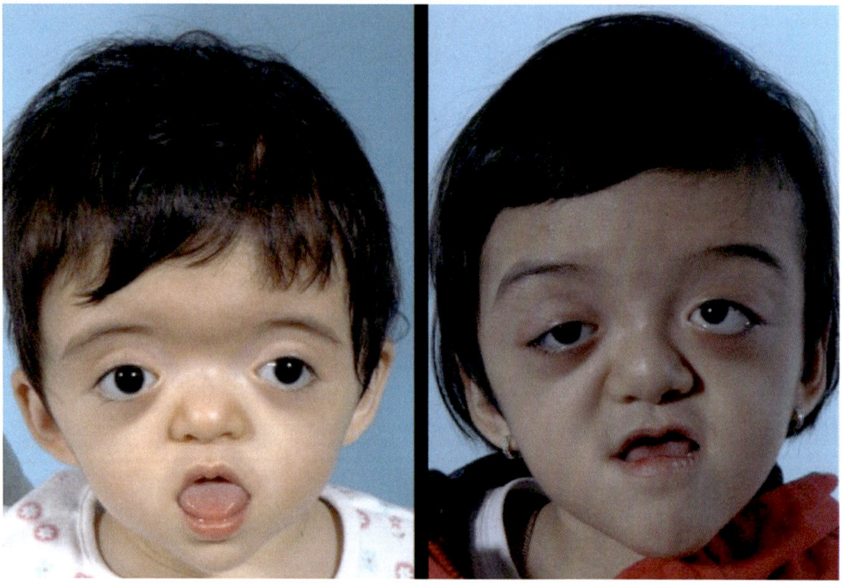

Apert patient before and after monobloc and facial bipartition at age 5.

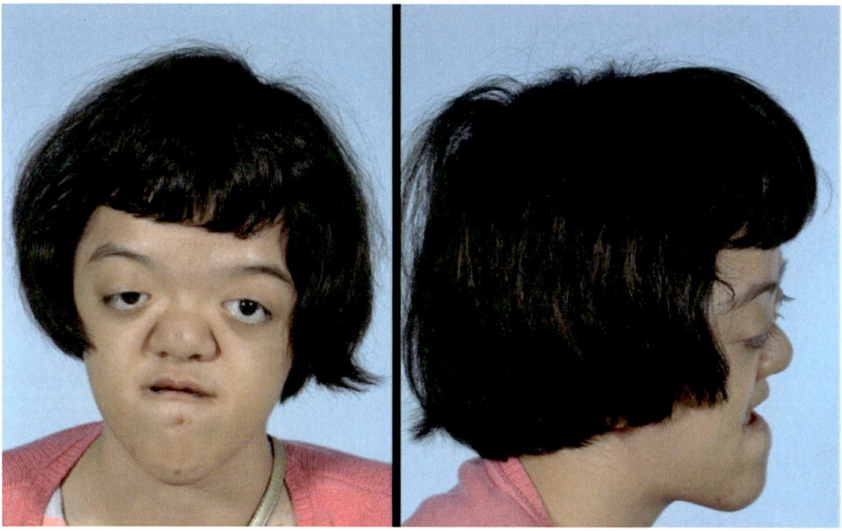

In mid-teens there has been no further maxillary growth, she was treated with a Le Fort 3 advancement using a RED device (Rigid External Distractor).

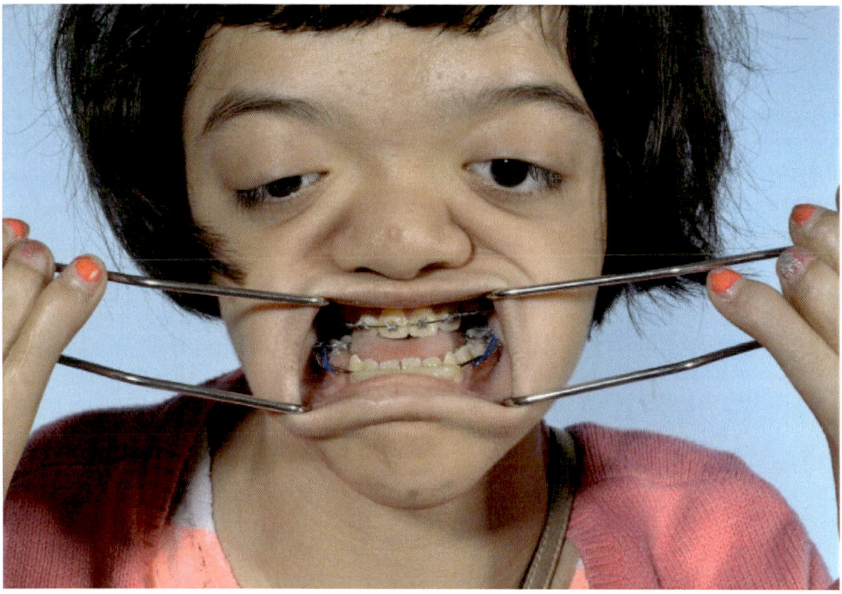

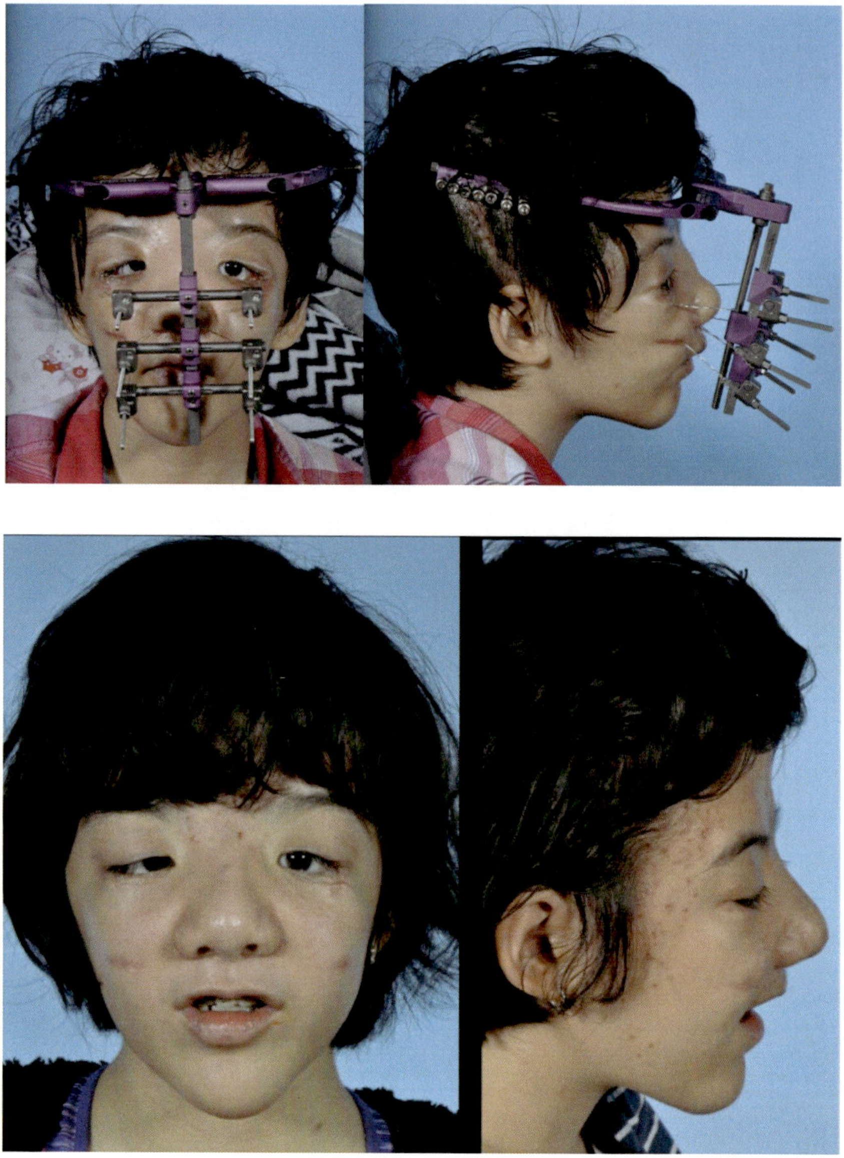

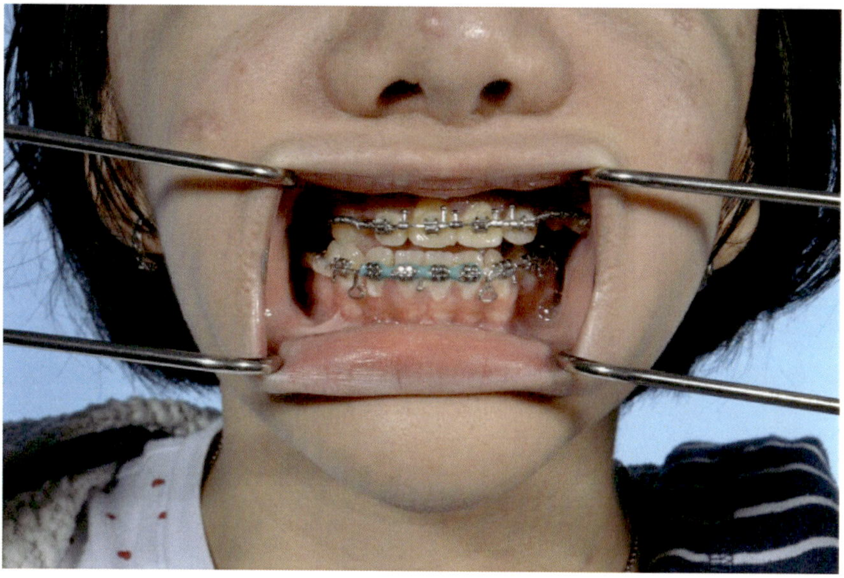

Juin 97 – PARIS –   LE CONGRES SUR LES D.O.G PROCESSES

Beaucoup plus intéressant que prévu

Sur les 88 présentations, 16 ont été très instructives bien que j'e
trentaine de bonnes. Du 7% c'est exceptionnel.

Satisfaction ou amertume ? Dix-huit fois (18) des projets -T- élab
ont été démontrés ou évoqués. En Décembre 96 ils étaient prêts à
Freiburg avec 20 ou 30 autres, pas tous réalisables. Plutôt que d
trou comme la CEPH-20, je les ai tous passés à Henry K.

Juin 97 – PARIS –   REFLEXIONS APRES LE CONGRES D.O.G. PR

1- "Régénérat" excellent mot, du moins en français, de même que
du régénérat" indique sa transformation histologique et mécan

T-6-20 2- La mesure des forces ?
On en est toujours au même point .... mort
TOTH avait annoncé ....
MOLINA avait annoncé ....
MALEVEZ (059) annonce 300g sur un elastic band et masque
KUNG (055) annonce 900g sur un palatal expander et 400g el
de Delaire
LOSKEN (082) annonce entre 15 et 50Kg sur le crâne du lapi
Or depuis deux siècles il existe des dynamomètres et des "ga

T-4-4 3- Monopin ou Twinpin ?
Henry-K comme David-M et les deux Fernando pensent que le
est suffisant pour la D.O.G. des C.F.D.
Pourquoi pas des minipins croisées peut-être plus faciles à ju
parallèles ?

4- Monocortical (028) ou bicortical comme tous les autres pour la
Pourquoi pas monocortical comme sur la voûte ?
Pourquoi pas des PEGS monocorticales auto-perforantes (K.L.

T-4-6 5- Modifier la direction des Forces : le "VECTEUR"
Henry-K est de mon avis : la ROTULE (B.aS.) ou plutôt sa f
à cupules ouvertes ou bien les joints accouplés du type Clous
Ginestet déjà utilisés dans les anciens fixateurs externes, sur
sur le T.E.C.F. system

T-4-7 6- Modifier la direction des Forces : le "VECTEUR"
En ... j'ai déjà dessiné le S.S. Curved-Telescopic distractor
sieurs courbures
Pourrait-on modifier la courbure d'un Endo-Dis courbe enfant
C'est peu probable
Peut-on modifier la courbure d'un Exo-Dis courbe ?
C'est inutile puisqu'il suffirait de le faire tourner autour d'un

7- Comment -sur la mandibule - changer la direction des forces
En utilisant des flexible rods sur un Exo-Dis. Mais n'est-ce p
rétrograde nous ramenant au distracteur externe et utilisable
la mandibule

T-4-15 8- La glène des O.M.D. ?
Avec Tony j'ai vu deux cas (different paper) où l'épiphyse s'

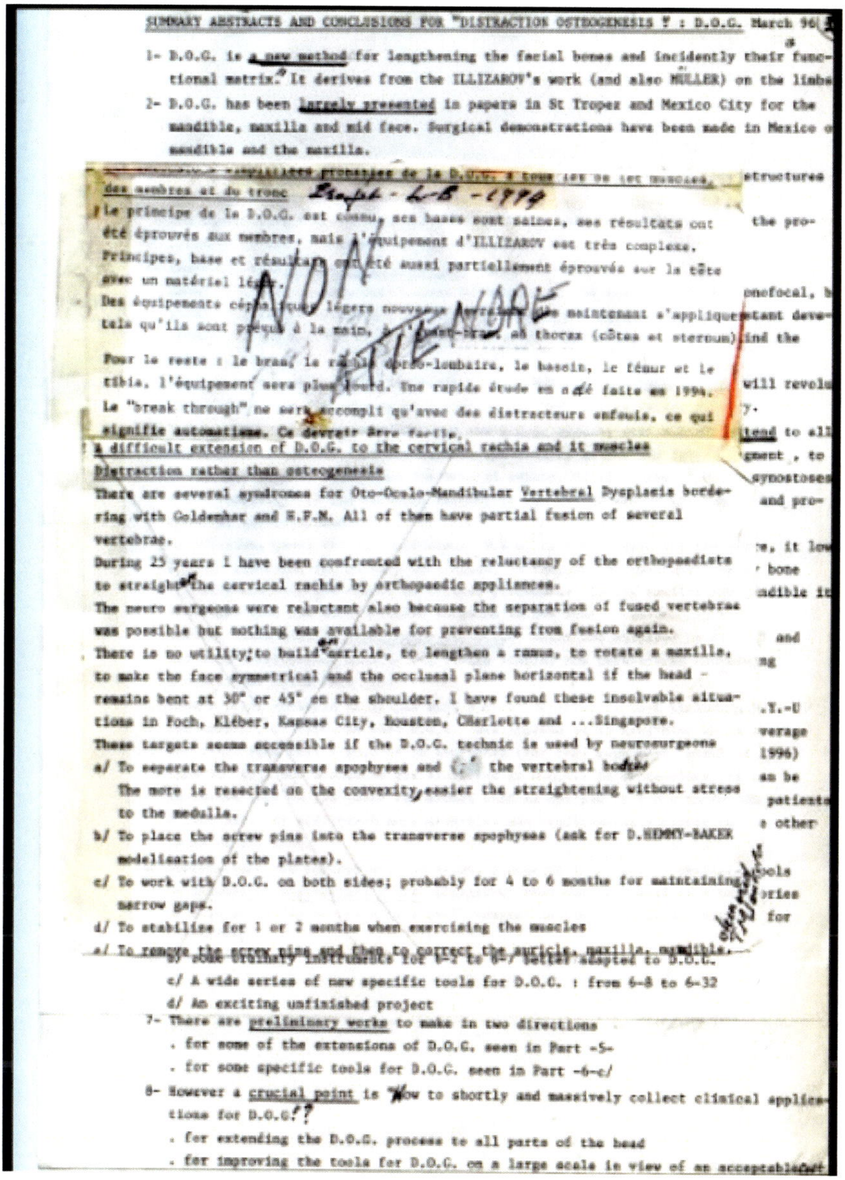

SUMMARY ABSTRACTS AND CONCLUSIONS FOR "DISTRACTION OSTEOGENESIS" : D.O.G. March 96

1- D.O.G. is a new method for lengthening the facial bones and incidently their functional matrix. It derives from the ILLIZAROV's work (and also MÜLLER) on the limbs

2- D.O.G. has been largely presented in papers in St Tropez and Mexico City for the mandible, maxilla and mid face. Surgical demonstrations have been made in Mexico [illegible] mandible and the maxilla.

des membres et du tronc

Le principe de la D.O.G. est connu, ses bases sont saines, ses résultats ont été éprouvés aux membres, mais l'équipement d'ILLIZAROV est très complexe. Principes, base et résultats ont été aussi partiellement éprouvés sur la tête avec un matériel léger.

Des équipements [illegible] légers nouveaux [illegible] maintenant s'appliquer tels qu'ils sont presque à la main, [illegible] thorax (côtes et sternum).

Pour le reste : le bras, le rachis dorso-lombaire, le bassin, le fémur et le tibia, l'équipement sera plus lourd. Une rapide étude en a été faite en 1994. Le "break through" ne sera accompli qu'avec des distracteurs enfouis, ce qui signifie automatisme. Ce devrait être facile.

a difficult extension of D.O.G. to the cervical rachis and it muscles

Distraction rather than osteogenesis

There are several syndromes for Oto-Oculo-Mandibular Vertebral Dysplasia bordering with Goldenhar and H.F.M. All of them have partial fusion of several vertebrae.

During 25 years I have been confronted with the reluctancy of the orthopaedists to straighten the cervical rachis by orthopaedic appliances.

The neuro surgeons were reluctant also because the separation of fused vertebrae was possible but nothing was available for preventing from fusion again.

There is no utility; to build an auricle, to lengthen a ramus, to rotate a maxilla, to make the face symmetrical and the occlusal plane horizontal if the head remains bent at 30° or 45° on the shoulder. I have found these insolvable situations in Foch, Kléber, Kansas City, Houston, CHarlotte and ...Singapore.

These targets seems accessible if the D.O.G. technic is used by neurosurgeons

a/ To separate the transverse apophyses and [illegible] the vertebral bodies

The more is resected on the convexity, easier the straightening without stress to the medulla.

b/ To place the screw pins into the transverse apophyses (ask for D.HEMMY-BAKER modelisation of the plates).

c/ To work with D.O.G. on both sides; probably for 4 to 6 months for maintaining narrow gaps.

d/ To stabilise for 1 or 2 months when exercising the muscles

e/ To remove the screw pins and then to correct the auricle, maxilla, mandible.

c/ A wide series of new specific tools for D.O.C. : from 6-8 to 6-32

d/ An exciting unfinished project

7- There are preliminary works to make in two directions

. for some of the extensions of D.O.G. seen in Part -5-

. for some specific tools for D.O.G. seen in Part -6-c/

8- However a crucial point is how to shortly and massively collect clinical applications for D.O.G.??

. for extending the D.O.G. process to all parts of the head

. for improving the tools for D.O.G. on a large scale in view of an acceptable[illegible]

Distraction Osteogenesis: Tessier's thoughts about the Paris meeting on Distraction Osteogenesis

Tessier Classification, 1976

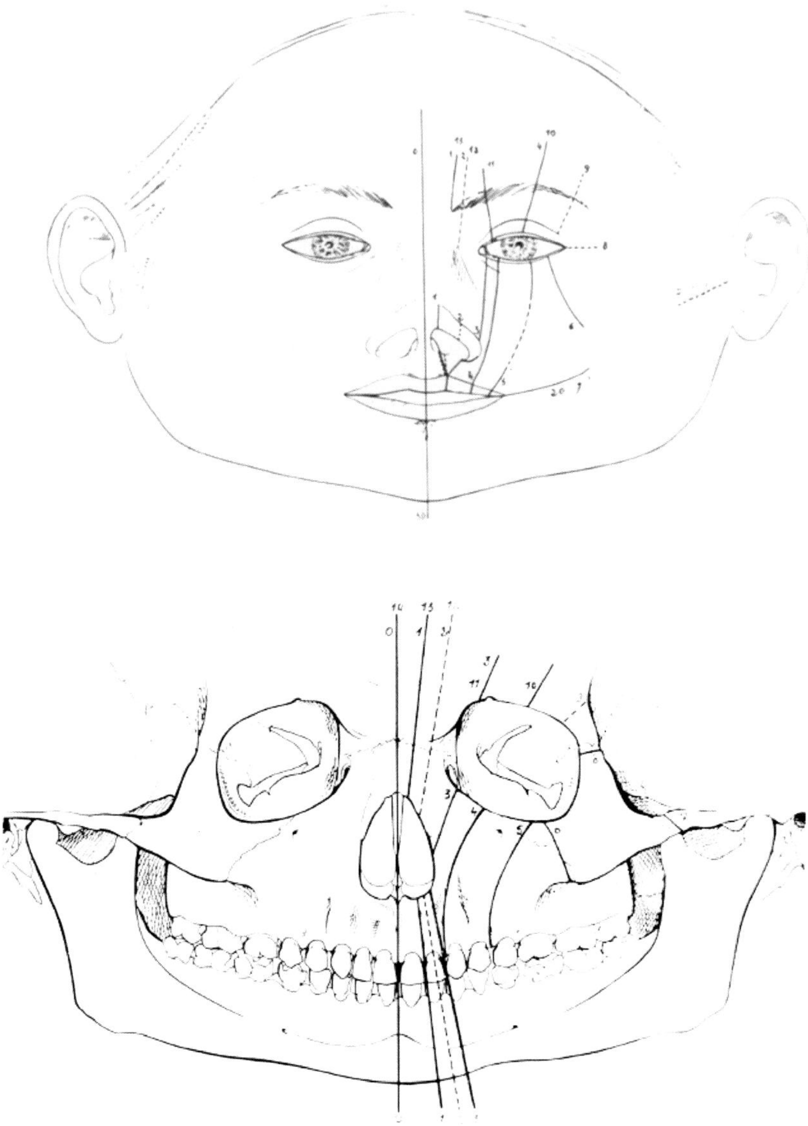

Tessier Clefts: Tessier Cleft Classification System

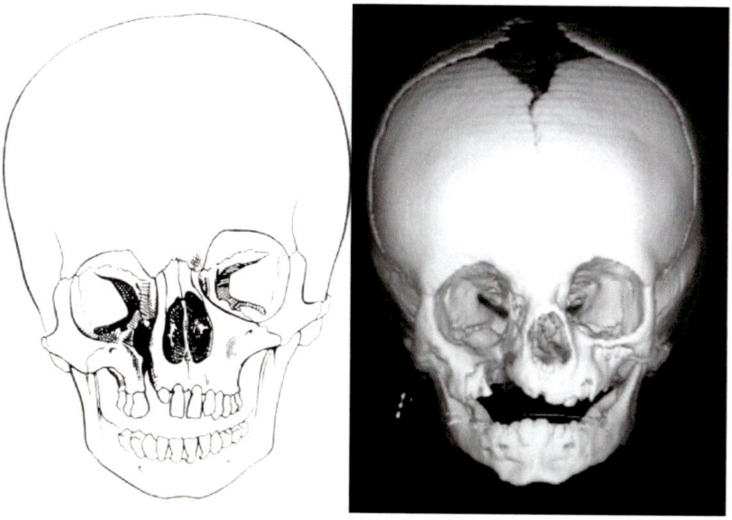

Tessier Clefts: A number 4 cleft. There is a septation between the nasal cavity and the maxillary sinus, making it easier to correct than a number 3.

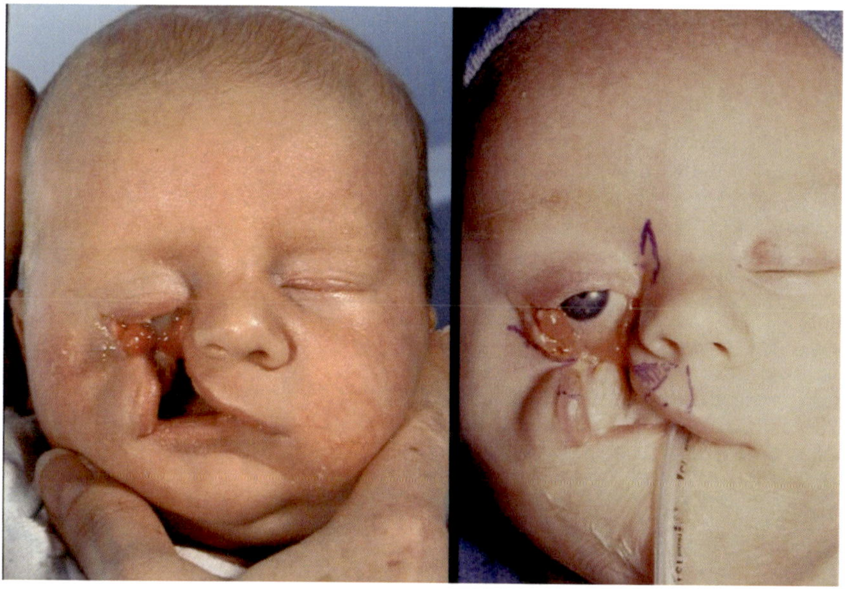

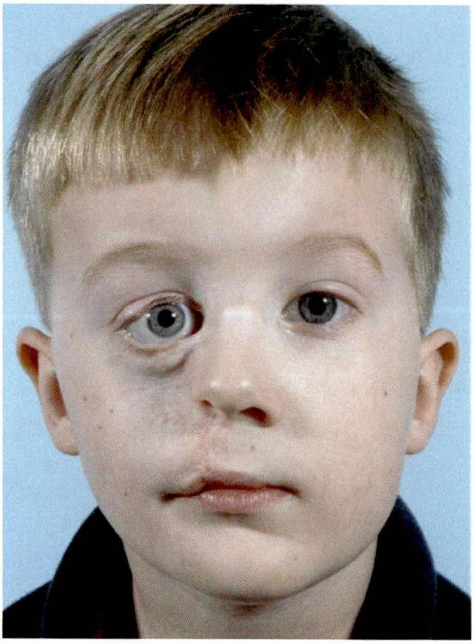

Good globe position but soft tissue deficiency of right cheek persists.

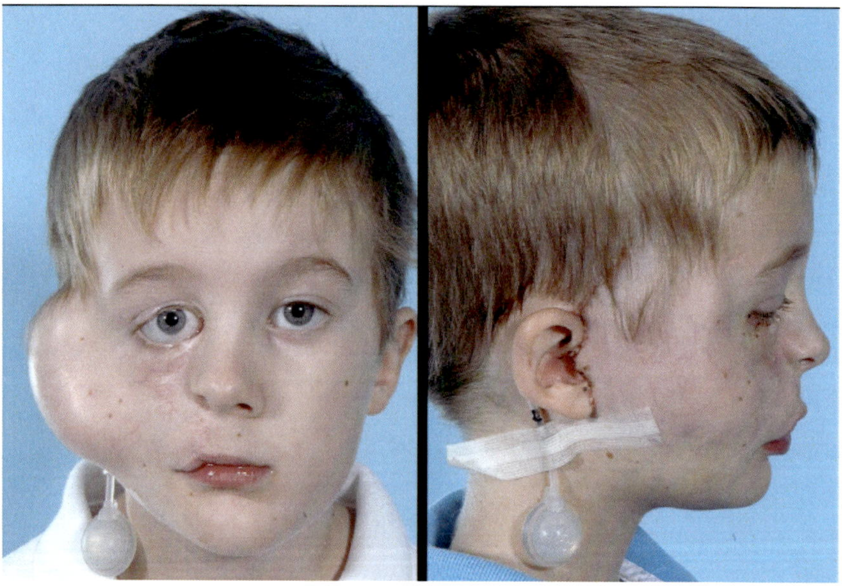

With tissue expander in place.

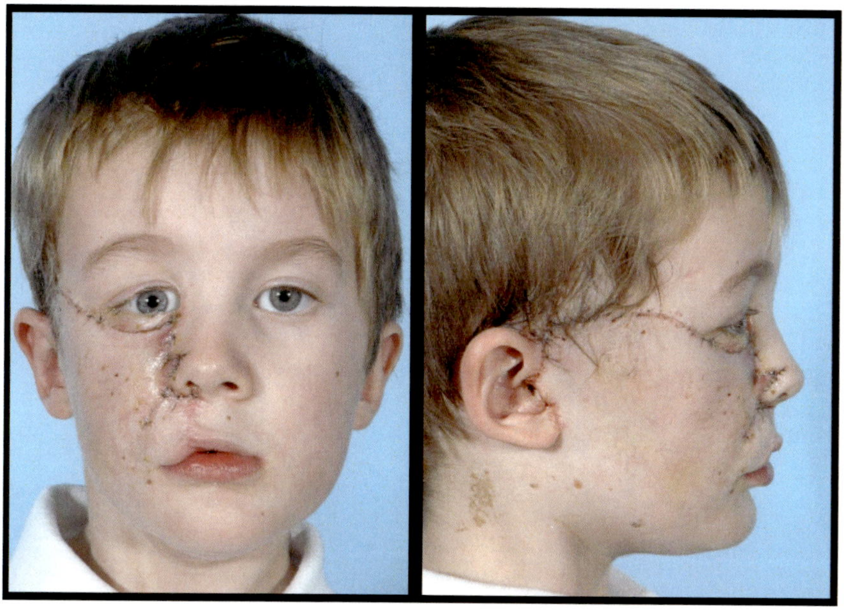

After tissue expansion of cheek to generate more soft tissue, globe position good.

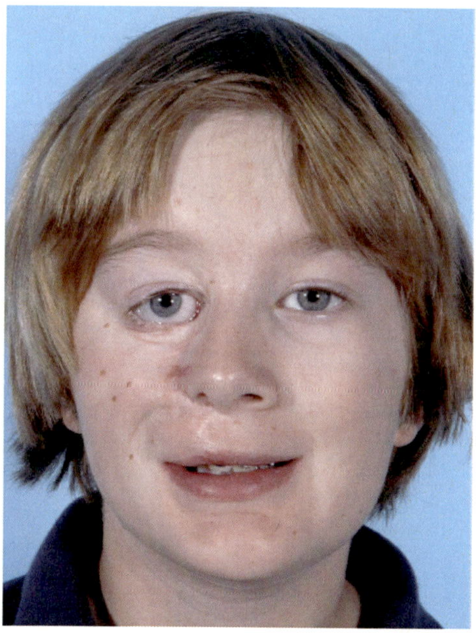

Now 14-years-old, 7 years after expander. Still has several millimeters of shortness of lower lid. A mid-face lift might correct this.

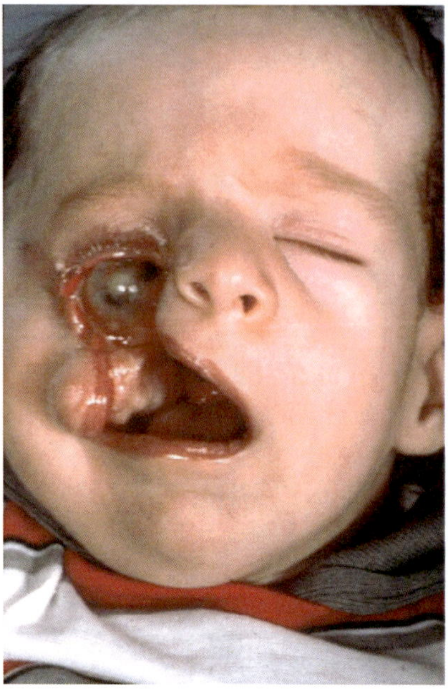

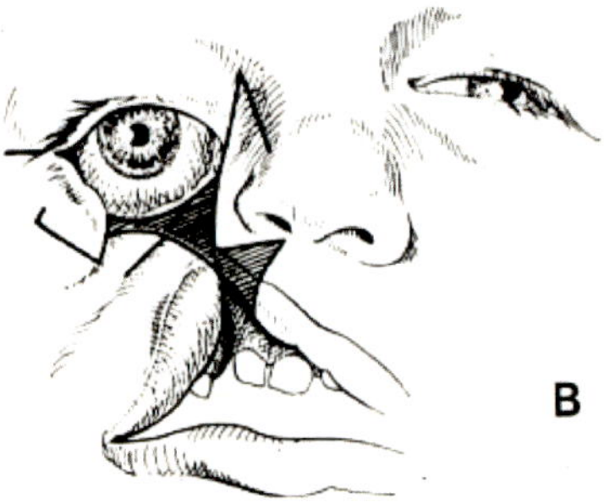

B

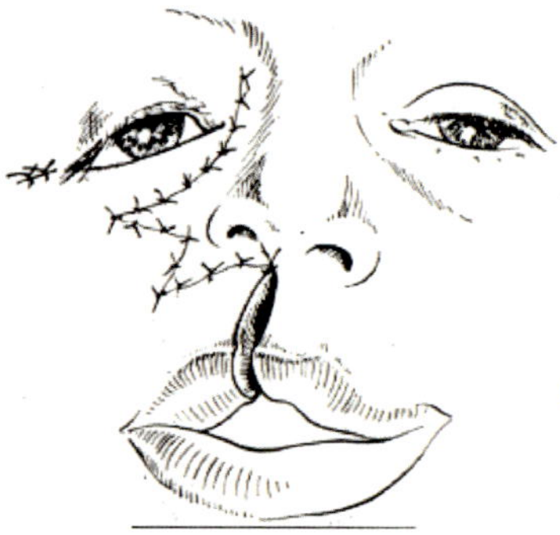

G

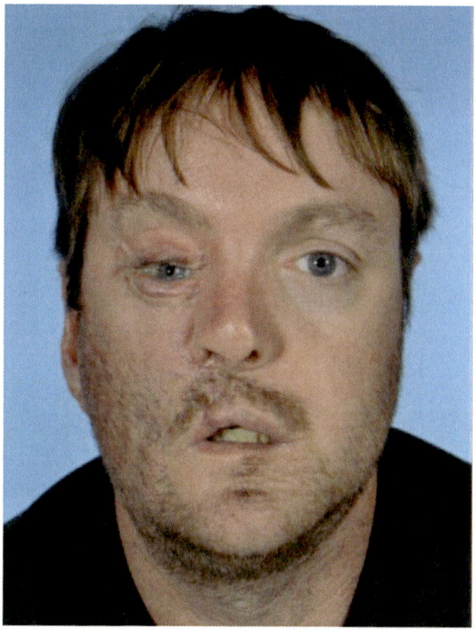

Another # 4 cleft with non-seeing eye which was maintained. 30-year result after multiple procedures. Bone graft placed secondarily at 1 year. Patient now drives a freight train.

Markings after Tessier. Rotation advancement for the lip, eyelid construction with vertical nasal flap, exposing area for transnasal blepharopexy, and advancement of lower eyelid flap. At the same time, full thickness calvarial bone graft to the orbital floor to prevent a vertical prolapse of globe into maxillary sinus and oral cavity. All done at 6 months of age.

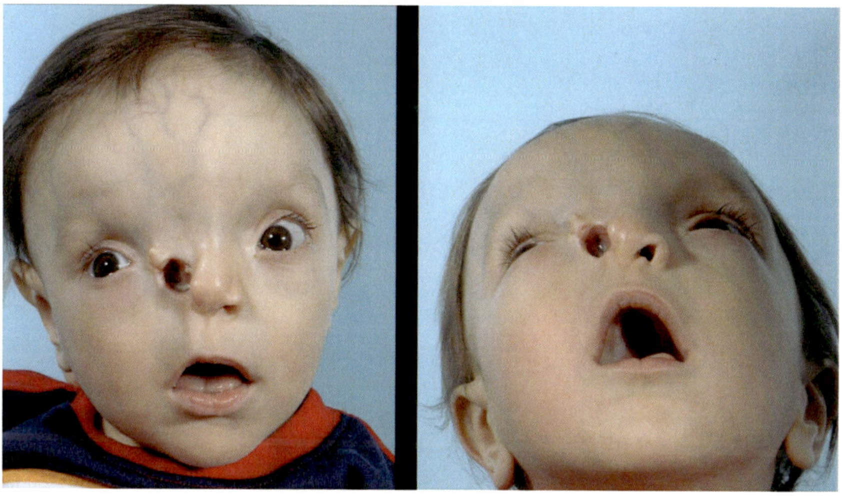

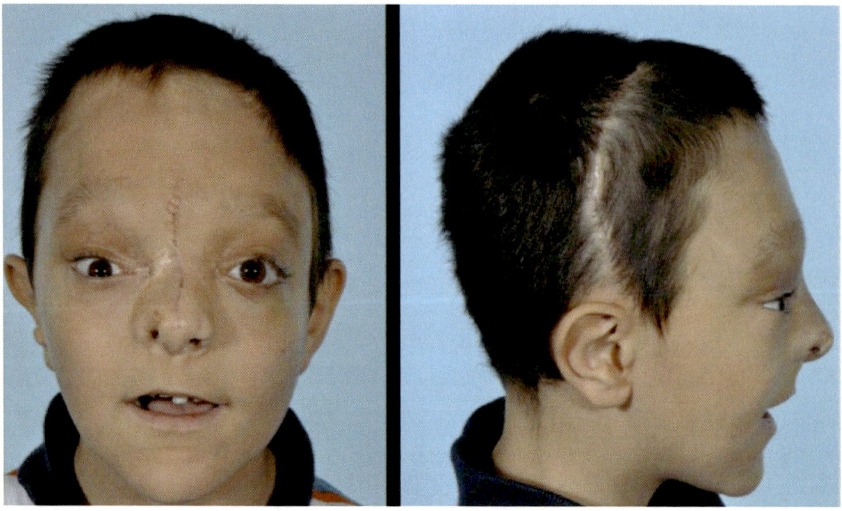

Tessier Clefts vs. Agenesis: I am uncertain whether this is a form of number 3 cleft or an agenesis. Patient treated with facial bipartition and turn-down flap of skin above nasal opening for lining and a forehead flap based on left post-auricular circulation.

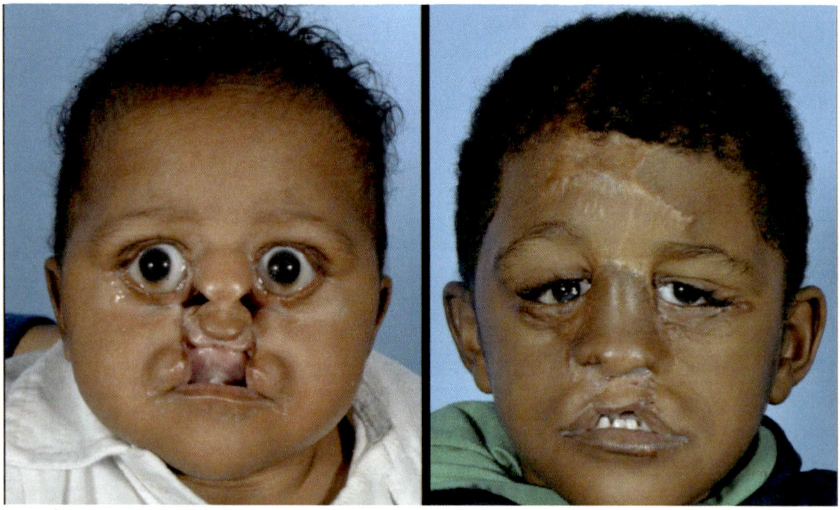

Atypical oro-ocular cleft: Atypical oro-ocular cleft with nostril opening almost at medial canthal level. Staged repair of the bilateral lip clefts and nasojugal flaps for lower eyelids with transnasal blepharopexy. Then after 6 months turn down of remnant of nasal skin for lining and posteriorly based forehead flap, midface lift and full thickness skin grafts for lower eyelids after a mid-face lift. There is a persistent posterior choanal atresia that will require correction.

Treacher Collins syndrome

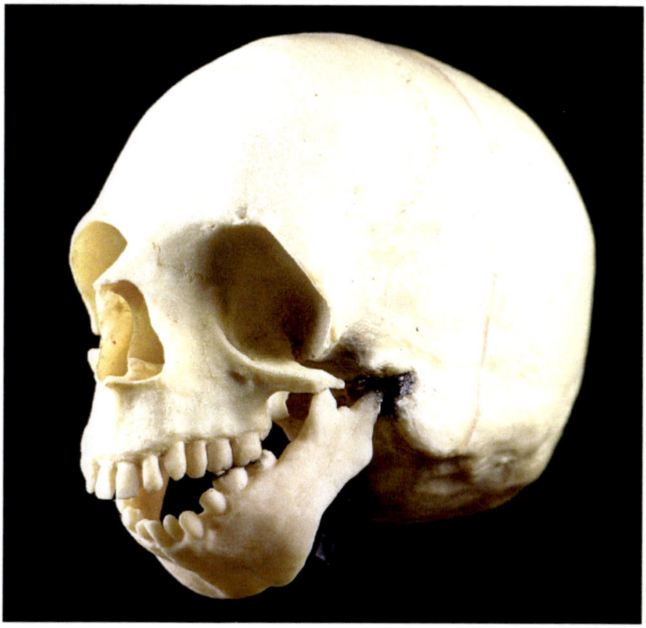

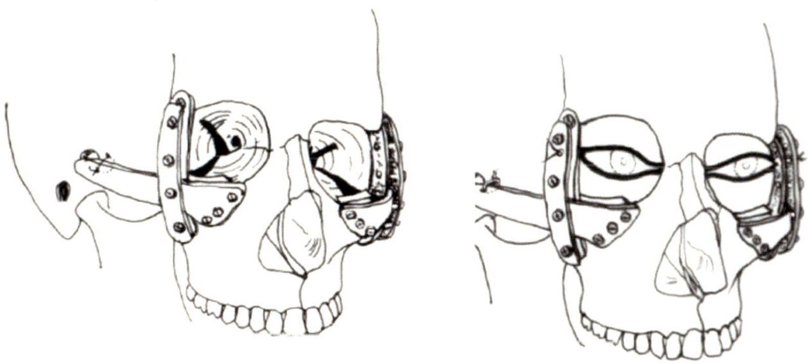

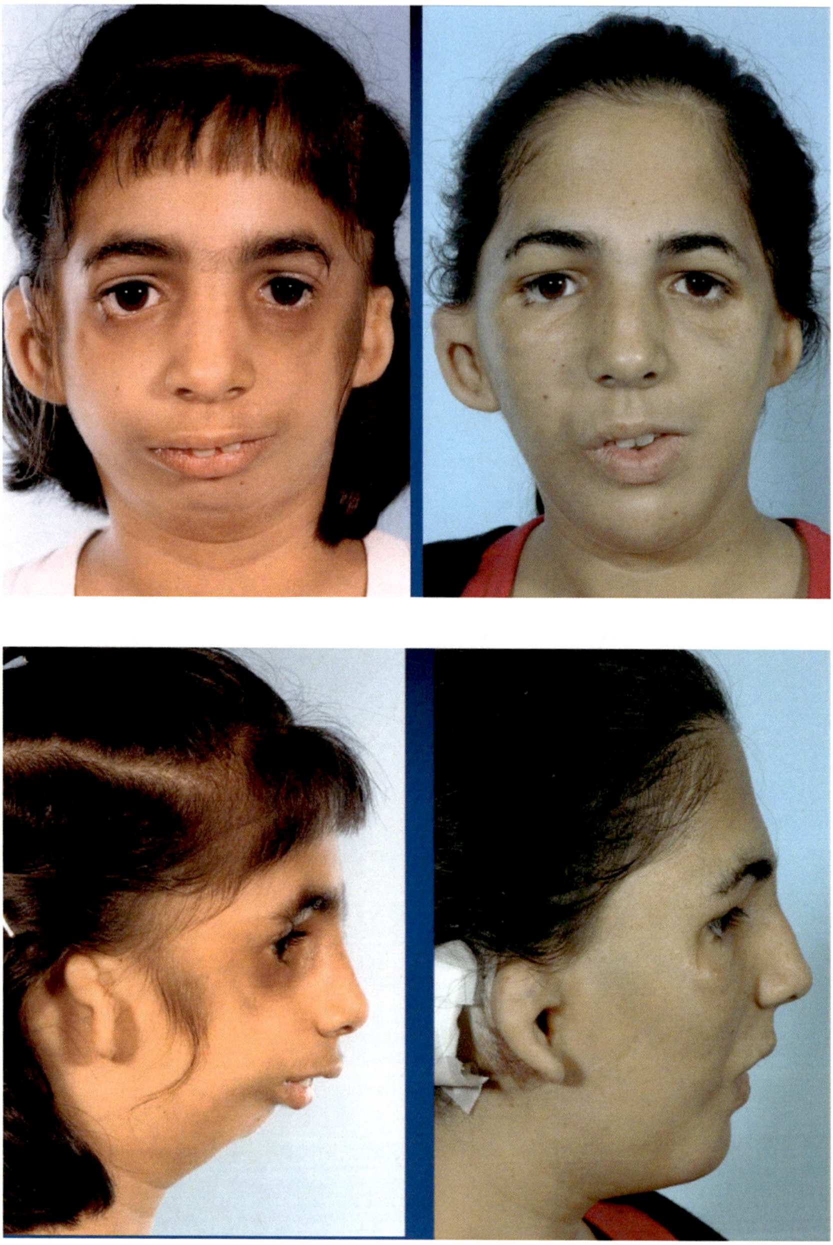

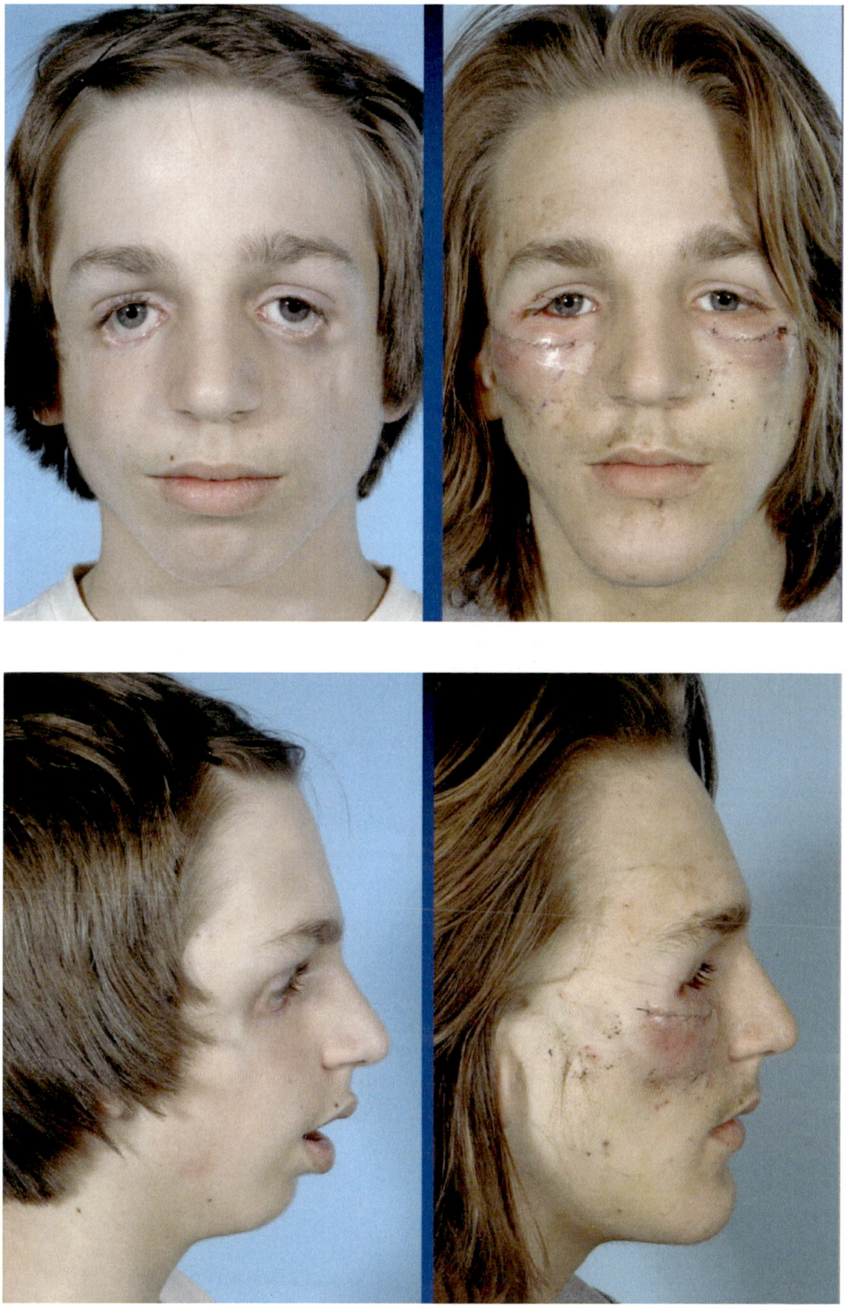

Use of the temporalis muscle

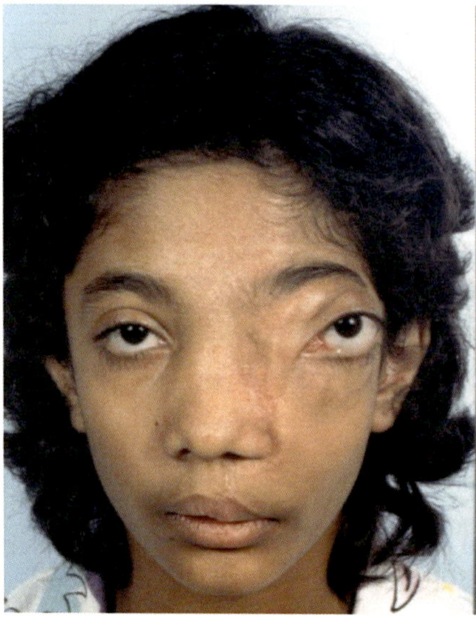

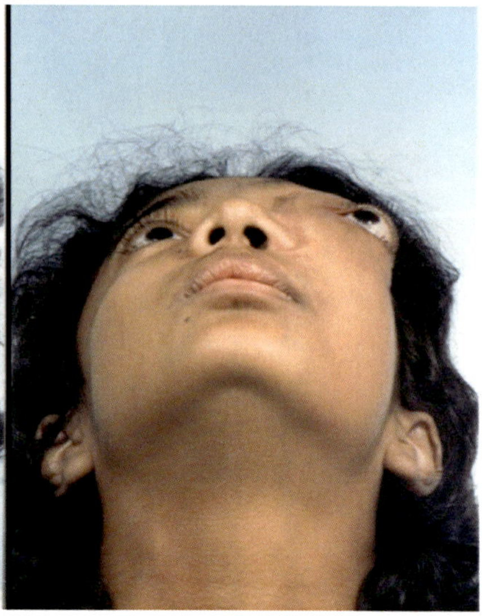

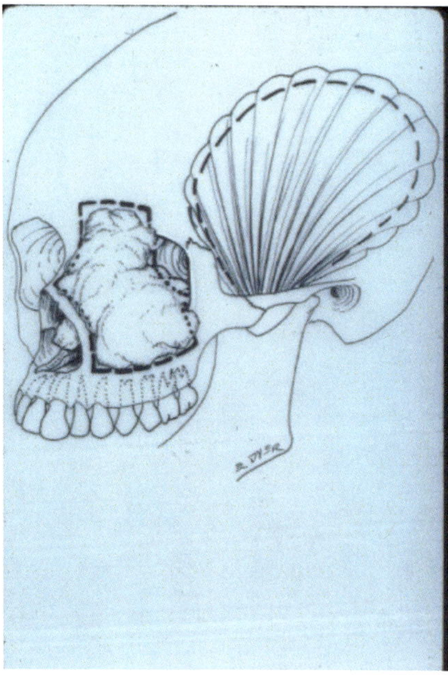

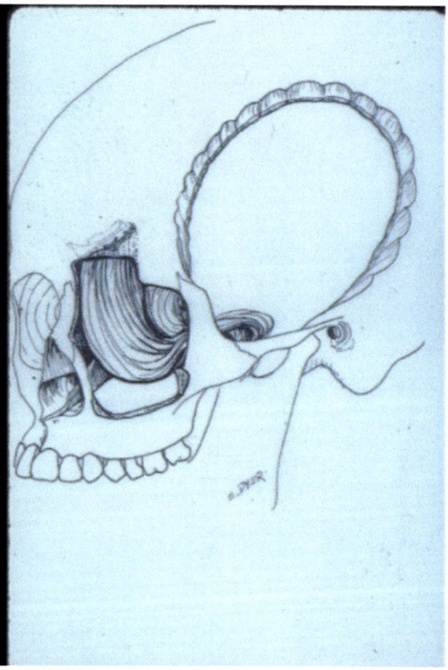

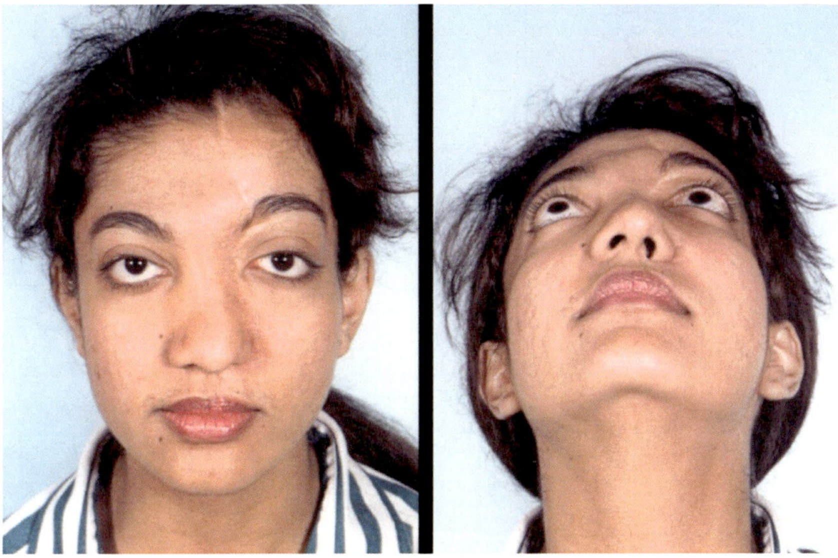

Fibrous dysplasia

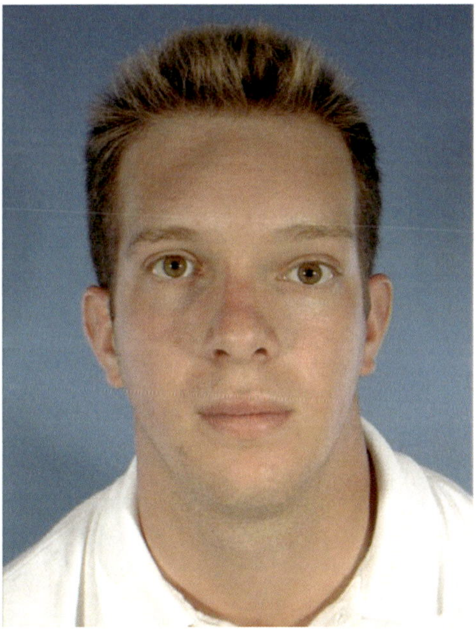

17-year-old with fibrous dysplasia (a benign slowly growing bone tumor) involving the entire left frontal bone and orbital roof with circumferential involvement of left optic nerve. In the supraorbital area the bone was over 5 cm thick.

Shown after resection of all involved frontal bone and prophylactic unroofing of optic canal, and reconstruction with split calvarial bone.

Shown one year and 8 years post-op with no recurrence and normal vision. Patient is now an orthopedic surgeon.

The use of split calvarial bone is another Tessier contribution. There is a large amount of bone available and the donor morbidity is minimal.

Prophylactic unroofing of the optic canal is controversial, but we feel it is preferable to waiting until there are irreversible visual changes and chronic compressive optic neuropathy.

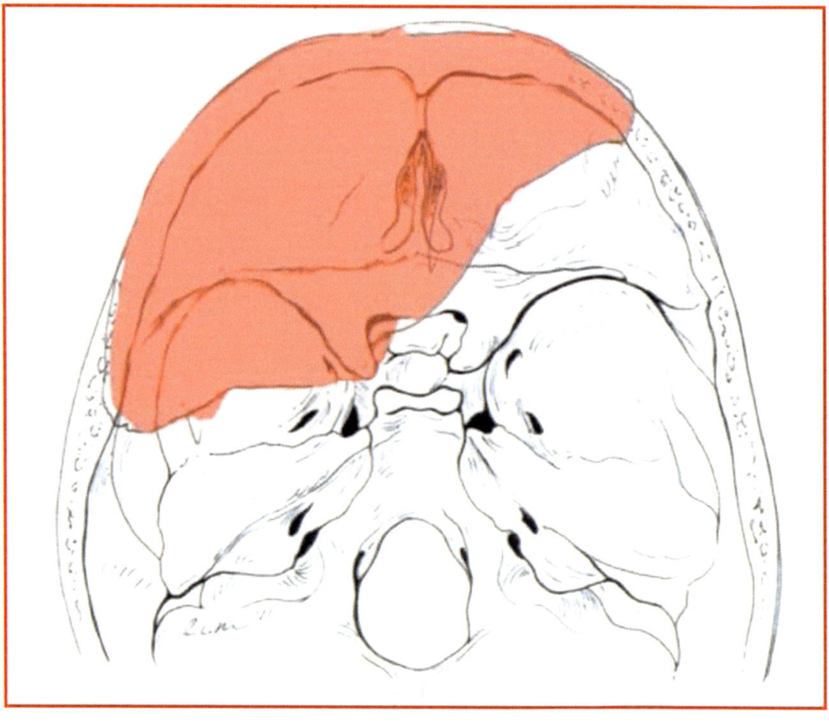

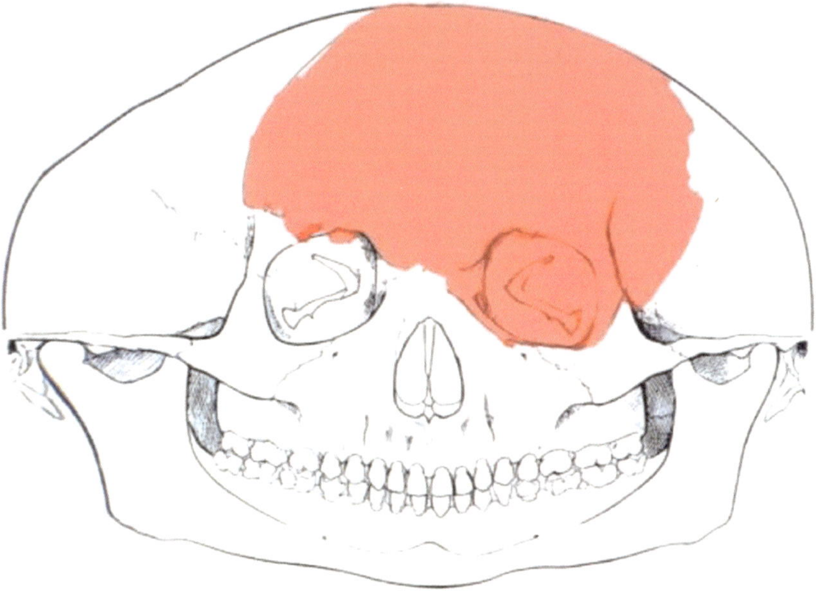

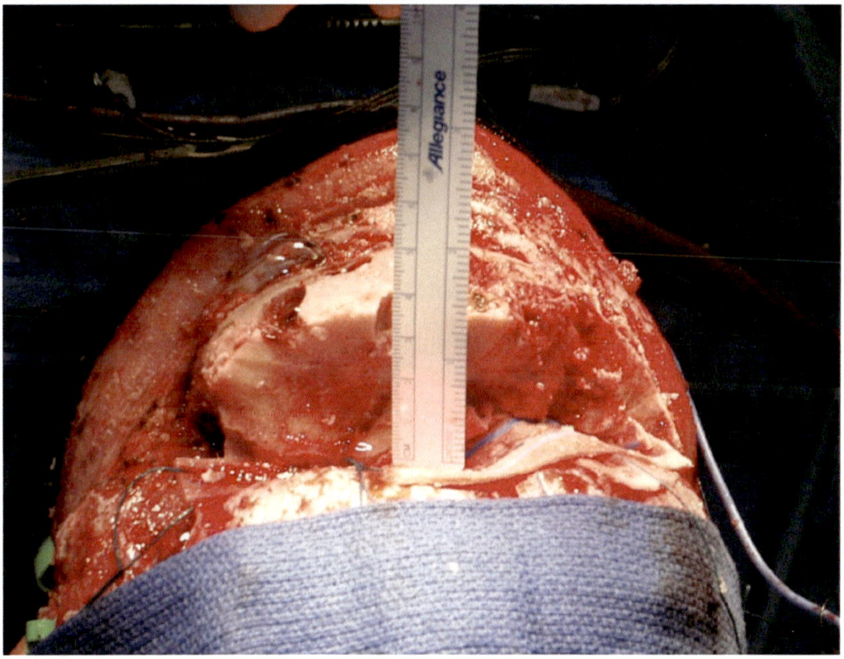
Allegiance

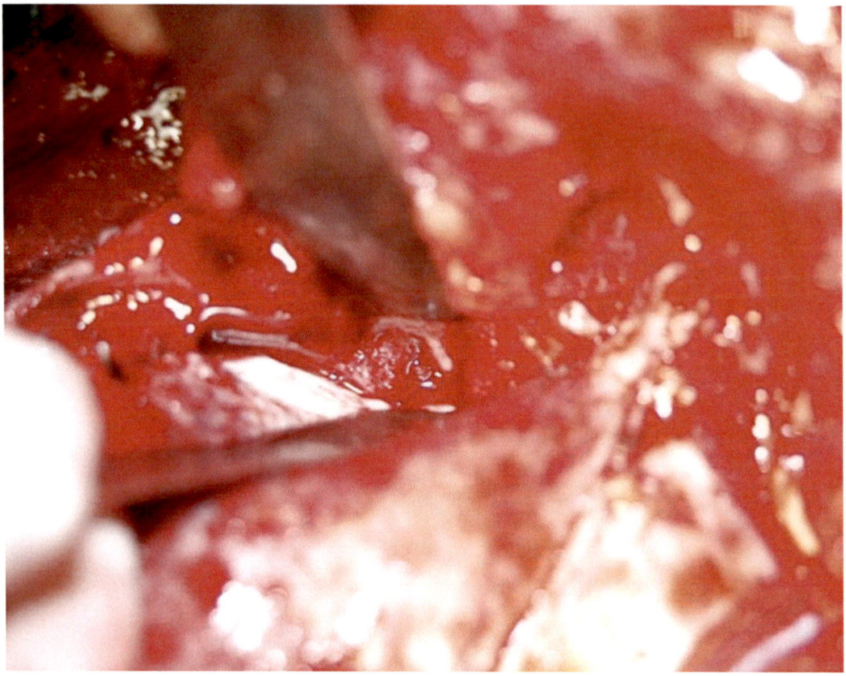

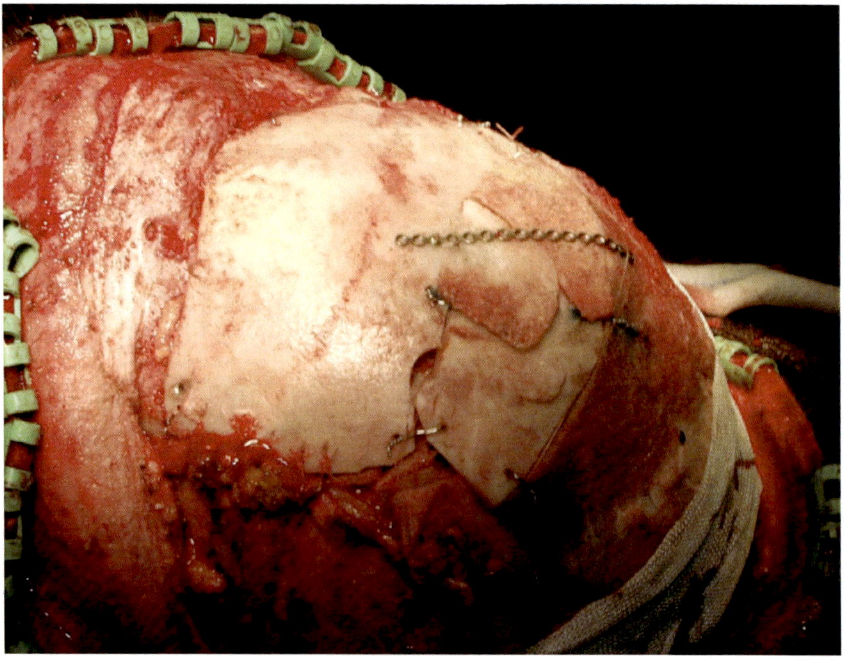

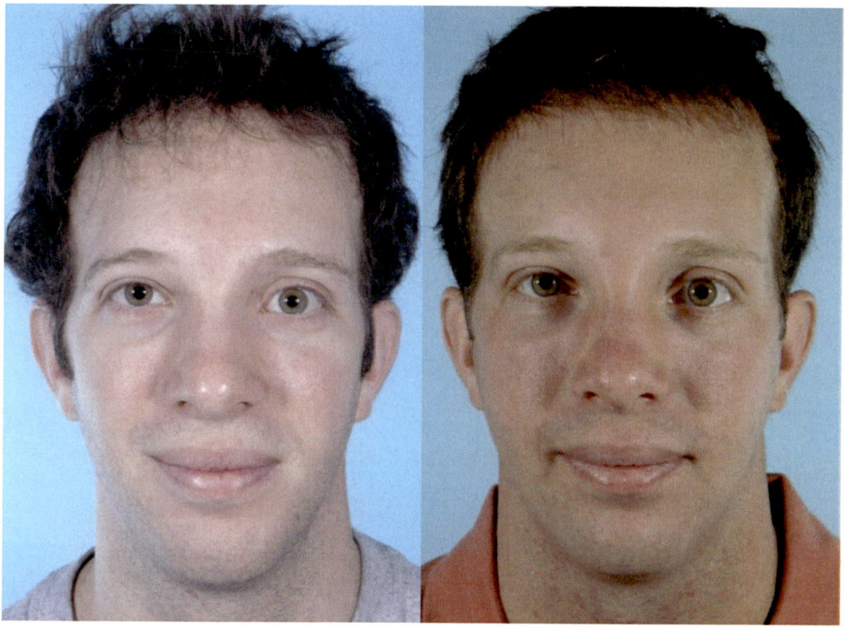

Impossible cases

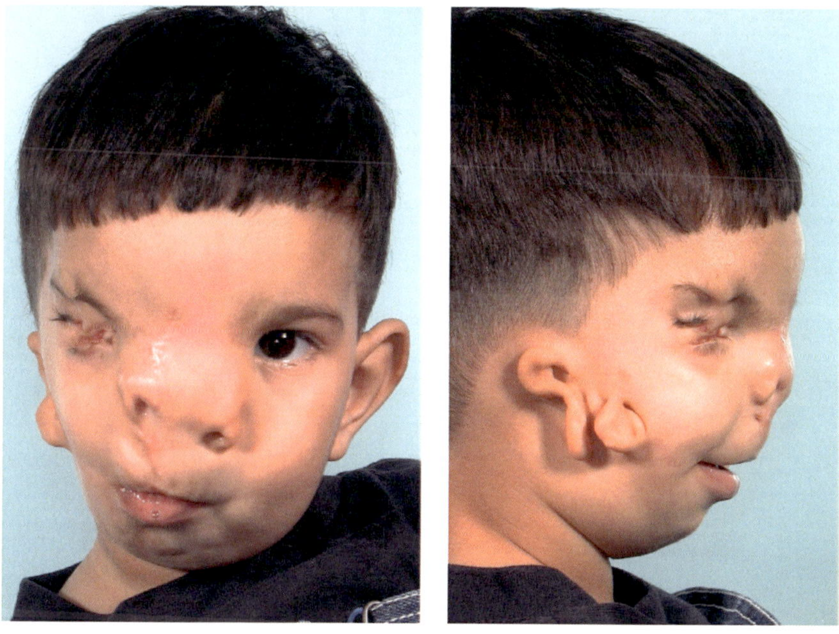

Case 1. Absent right hemimandible, orbit, and eyelids.

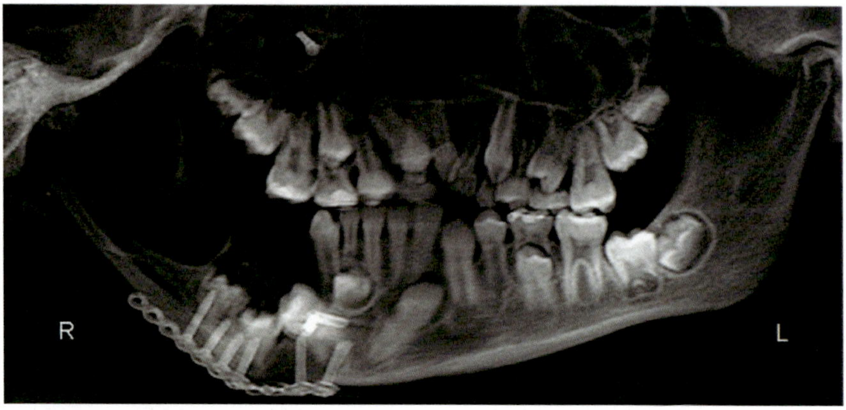

Panorex after rib graft for right mandible, good mouth opening.

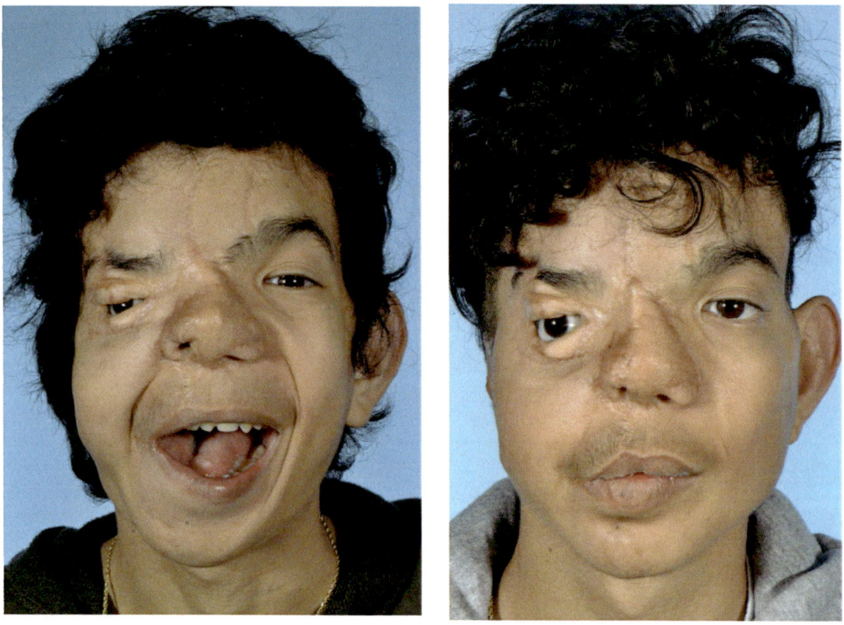

Almost finished, needs right lateral canthopexy and conchal cartilage graft with nasal revision. Wonderful kid who is entering college and wants to go into medicine.

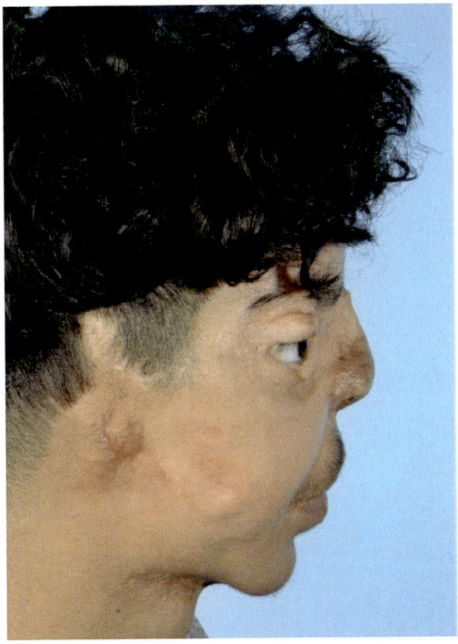

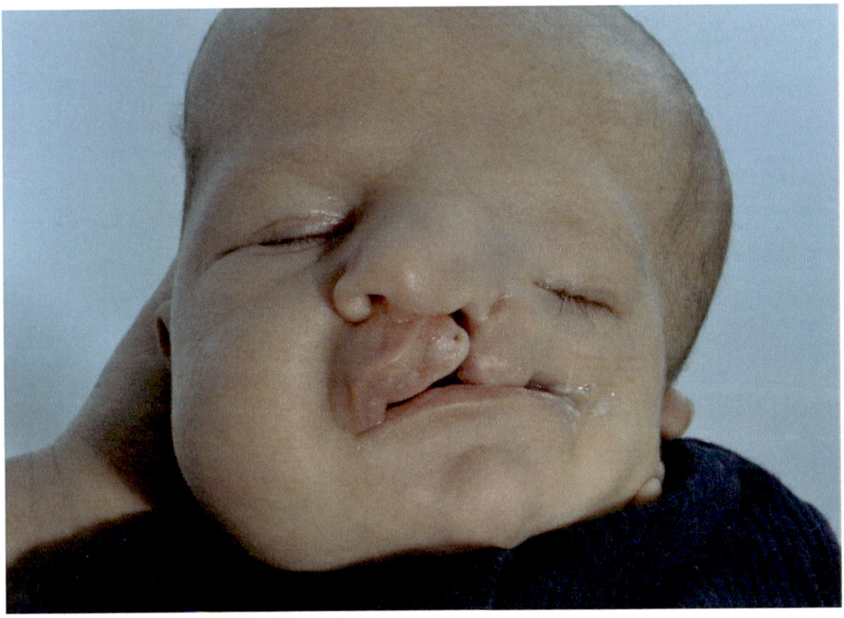

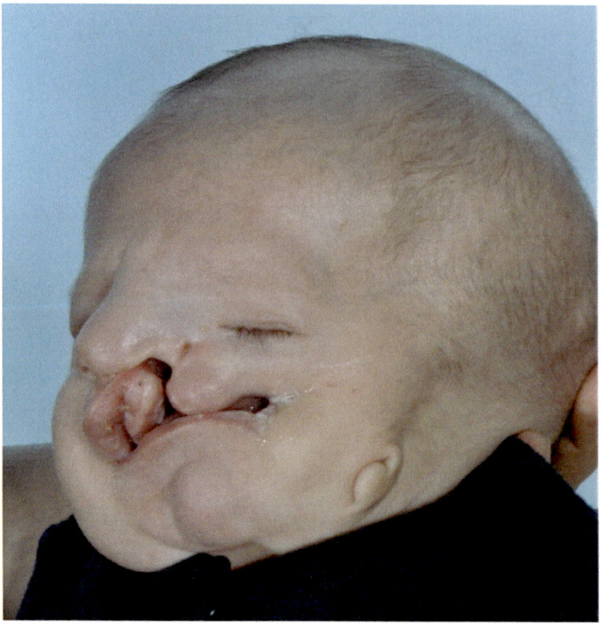

Case 2. Hemifacial agenesis: cleft of lip with virtually no face on left.

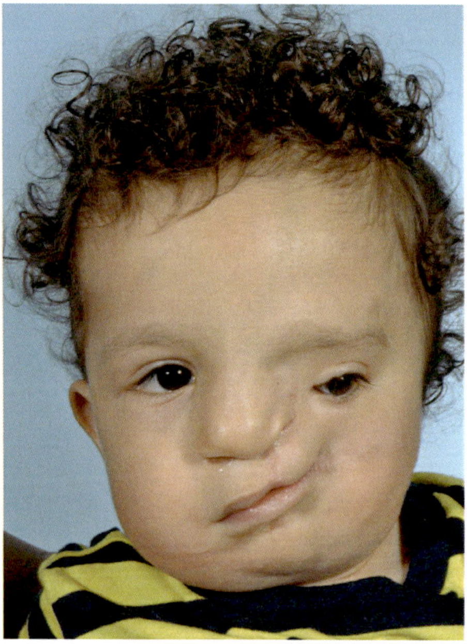

After closure of lip and 8 sessions of lipofilling left cheek and parasymphyseal area.

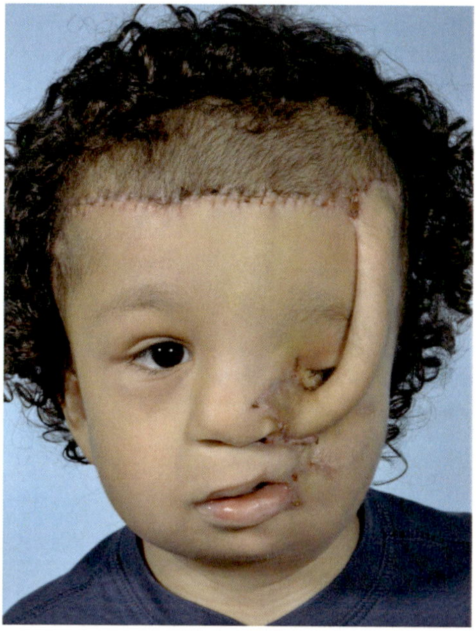

Tube pedicle fabricated from forehead after tissue expansion scalp and forehead.

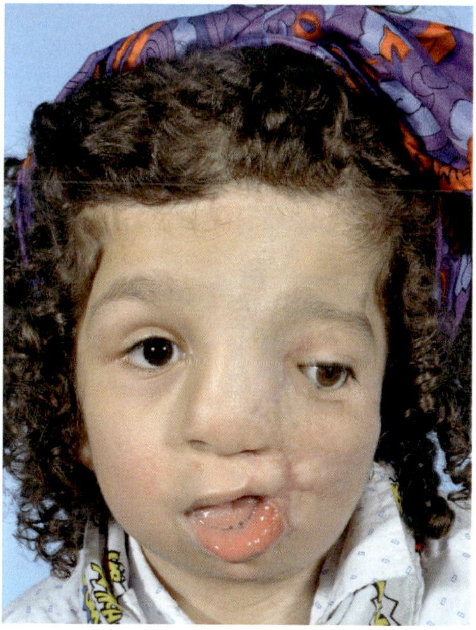

Current state awaiting further elevation left orbit with medial and lateral canthopexies.

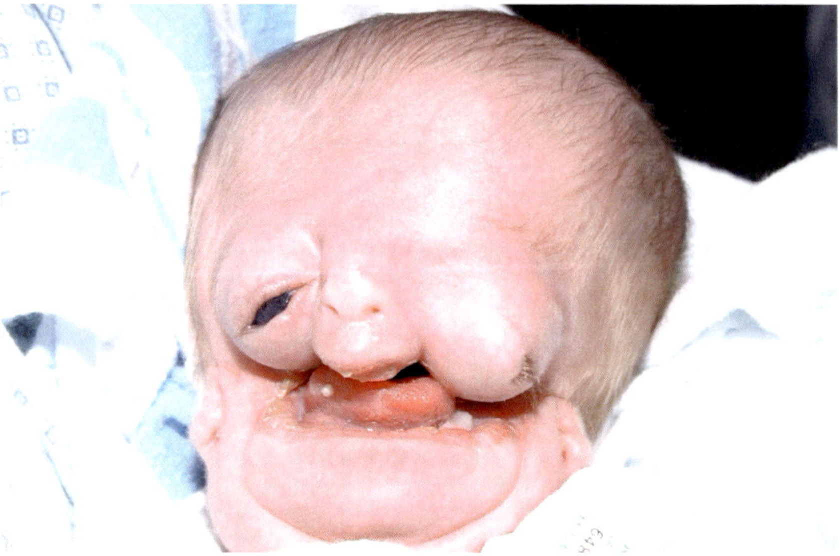

Case 3. Treacher Collins plus: Patient at birth with no midface and only central maxilla, there is a left eye present behind cryptopthalmic (fused) eyelids.

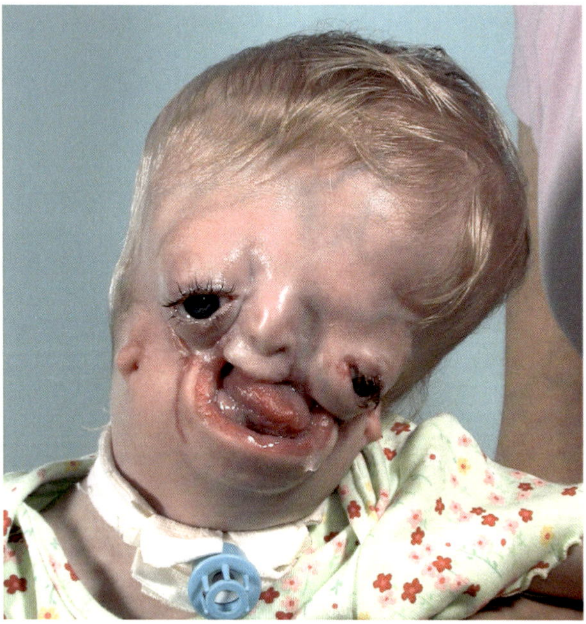

After opening fused eyelids over sighted eye, partial closure lateral facial clefts.

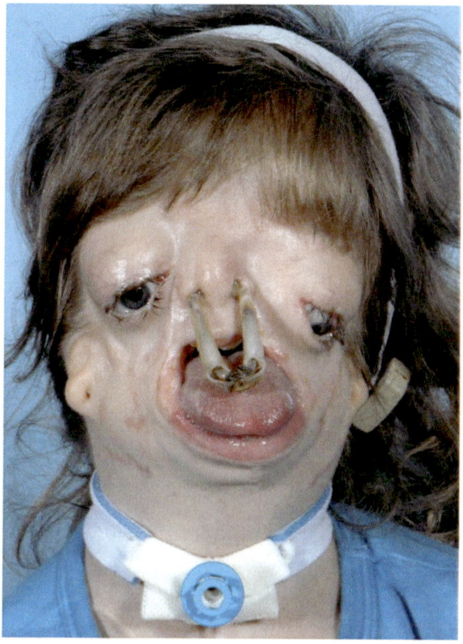

After creation of a nasopharynx via an intracranial approach followed by foreward and downward distraction of nasomaxillary segment, greatly increasing nasopharpyngeal space and making space for tongue.

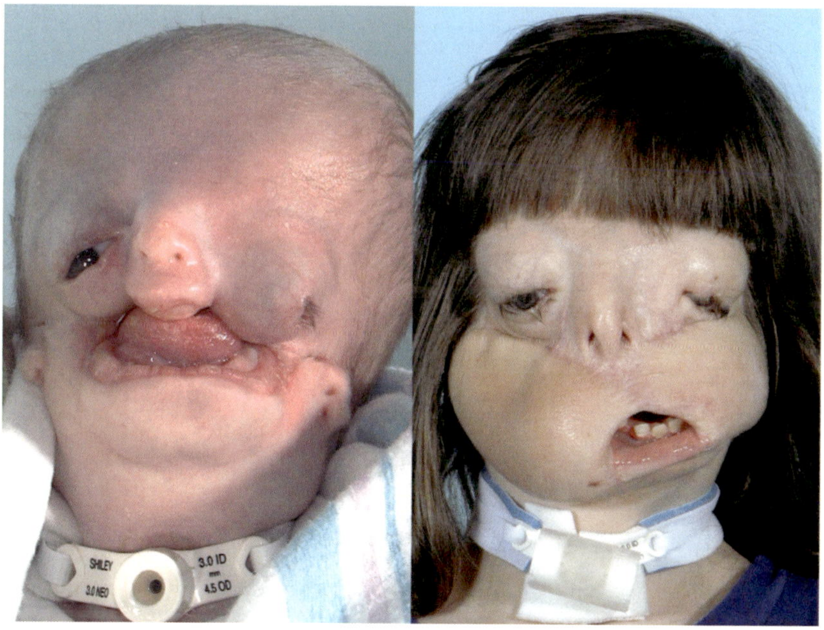

After transfer of two tube pedicles from posterior shoulder.

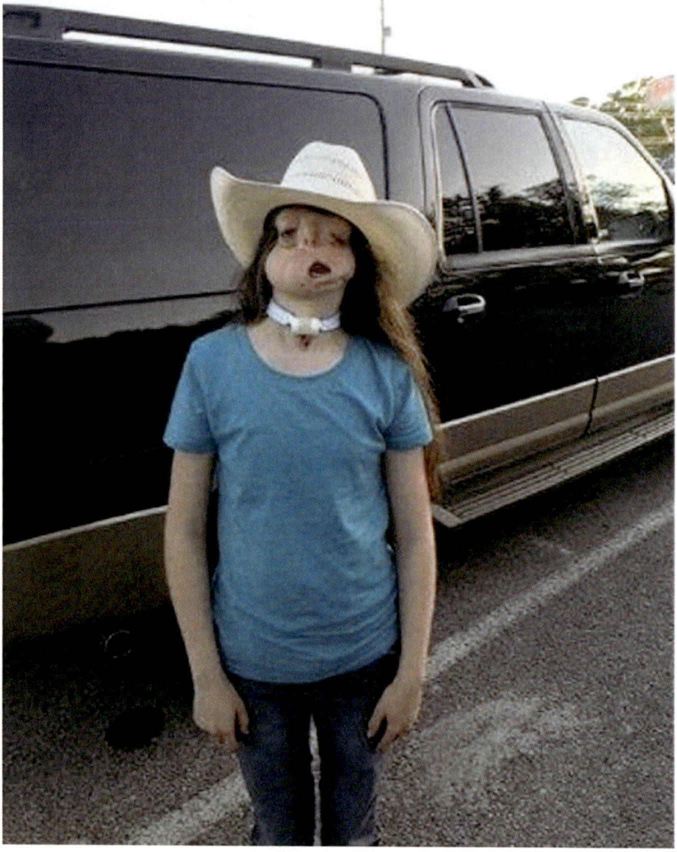

Patient at home in Texas. She can have further surgery if she wishes, probably would consist of debulking cheek flaps and making a nose with a forehead flap. This patient's story can be seen on the YouTube documentary, "Born Without a Face."

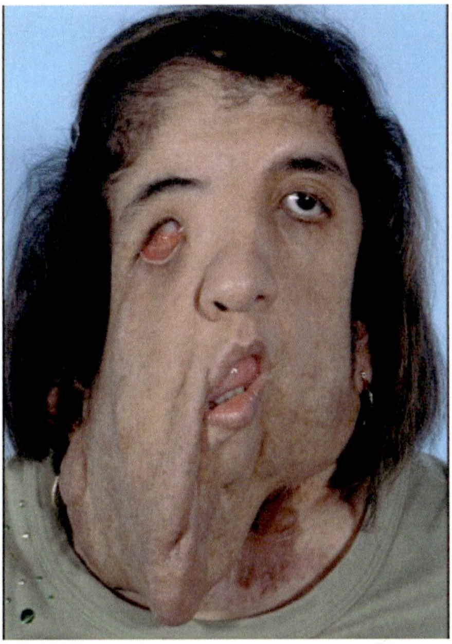

Case 4. Neurofibromatosis growing in right cheek has pulled right orbit down. The involved tissue cannot be resected and sutured since there is no dermis and the tissue needs to be replaced with healthy tissue.

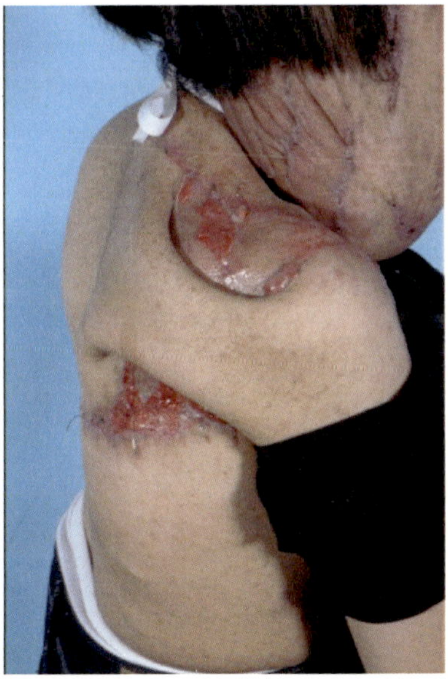

Fabrication of a tube pedicle on back of right shoulder. The skin graft could be removed after tissue expansion.

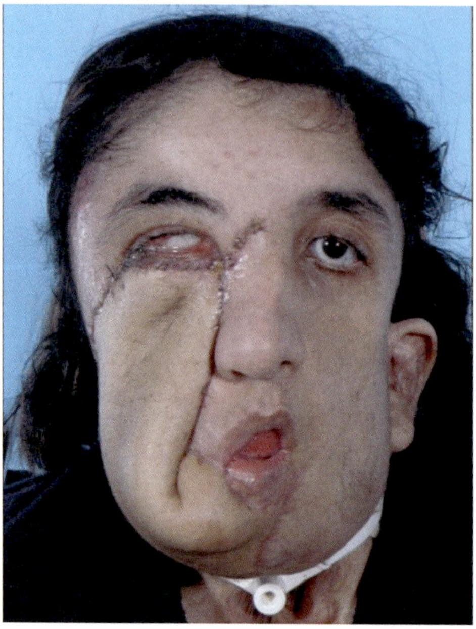

After transcranial elevation right orbit and waltzing up of tube pedicle.

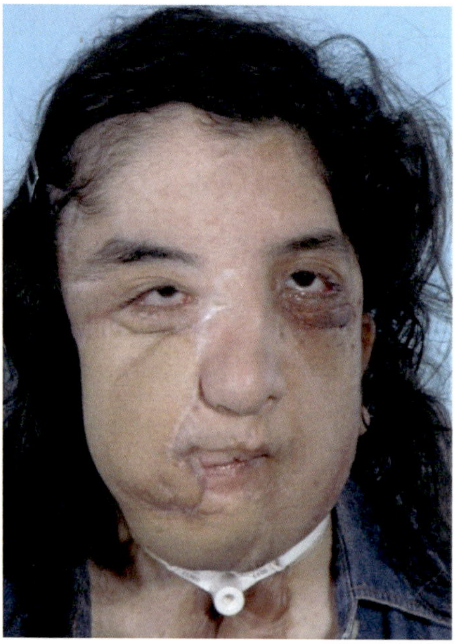

After further inset of tube pedicle, next step would be minor revisions and removal of tracheostomy.

Aesthetic Spinoffs of Craniofacial Surgery

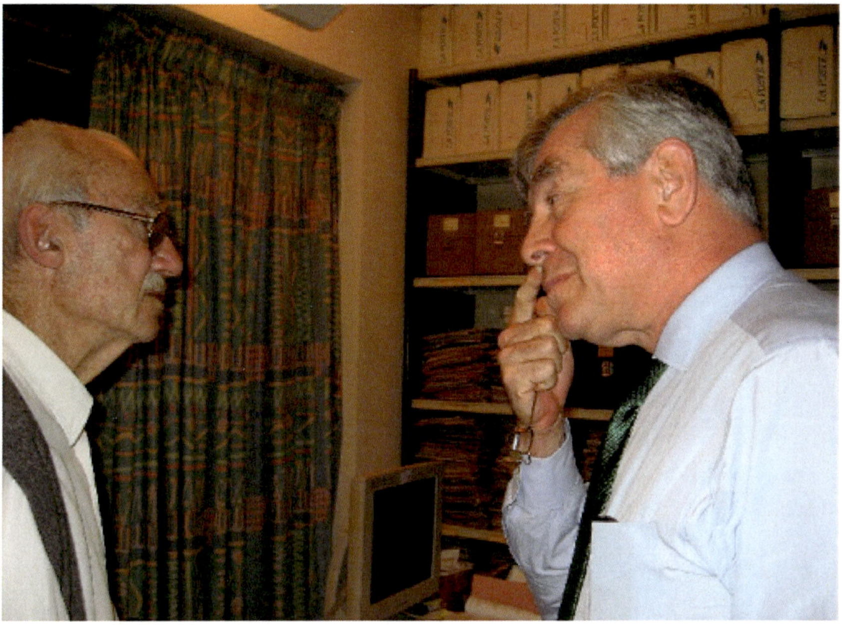

Dr. Tessier, not entirely jokingly, once asked me if I could do something about his turkey-gobbler neck. I said of course, he never came to surgery, but I corrected his neck (and mine) with the aid of PhotoShop.

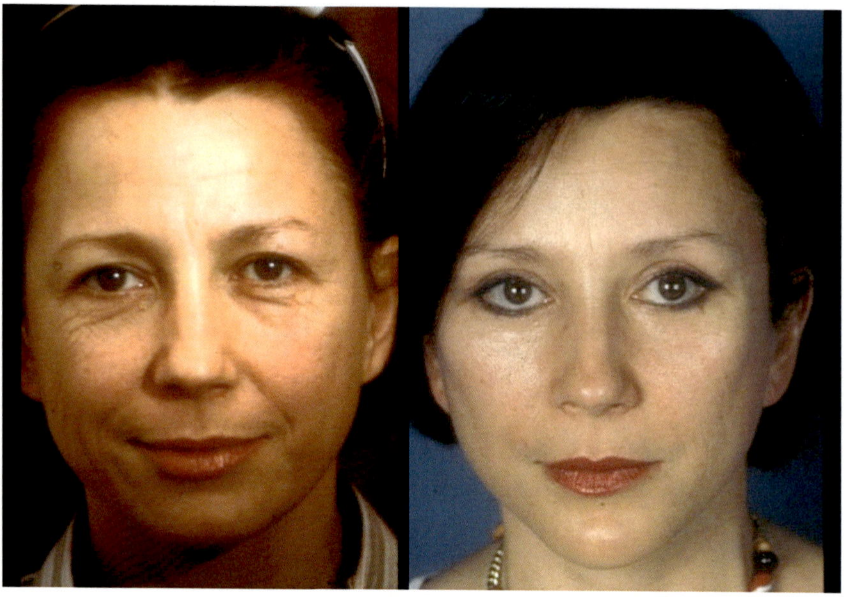

Darina Krastinova took over Dr. Tessier's Service at Hôspital Foch and was herself an expert on the "mask lift" or so-called subperiosteal facelift. Here she is shown after her own mask lift by Tessier, coronal dissection, forehead lift, contouring of lateral orbital rims, lateral canthopexies, malar bone grafts, minimal genioplasty and refinement of nasal tip, sub-SMAS facelift.

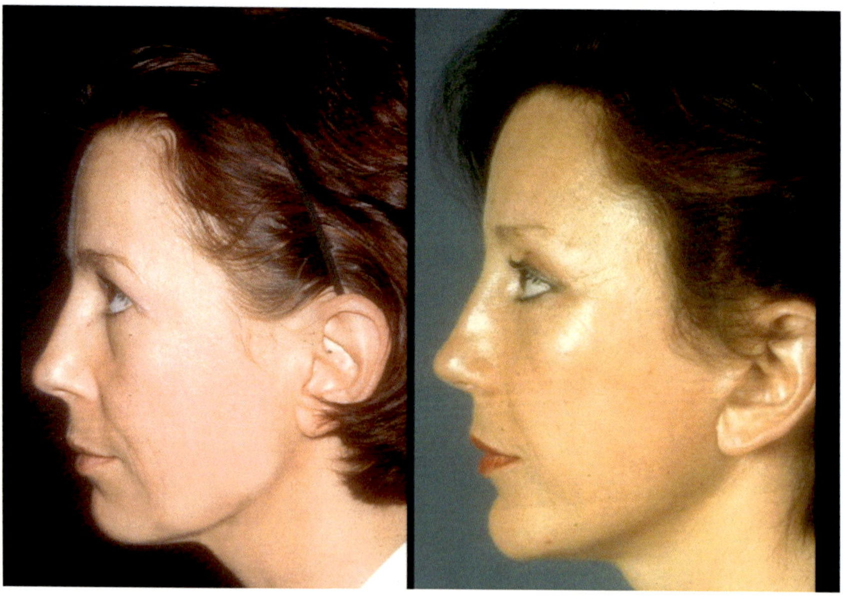

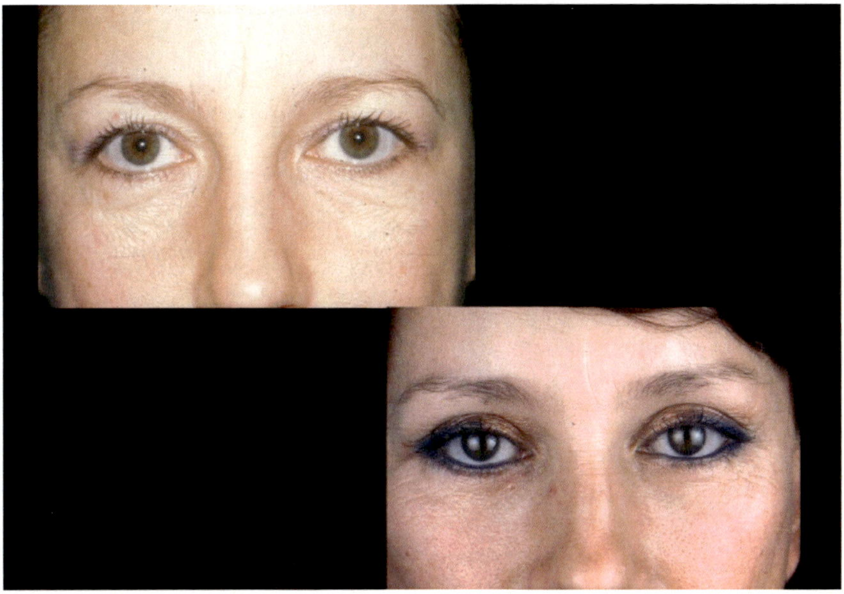

The SMAS

After hearing his friend Tord Skoog describe a superficial fascial layer in the face, in the mid-70's Tessier convened a group of young Parisian plastic surgeons to do anatomic dissections of this newly recognized structure.

Each team would take a different area: temporal, cheek, nose, neck. After completion of the dissection, all of the work was planned to be submitted to PRS as one paper.

Tessier had coined an acronym which would be the same in French and English: le Systeme Musculo Aponeurotique Superficiel, or Superficial Musculo Aponeurotic System, The SMAS.

One of the members of the team describing the structure in the cheek went ahead and sent their work in ahead of the others, contrary to the agreement. He has since gone on to claim that he is the "inventor" of the SMAS. This is false, and Tessier completely deserves the credit.

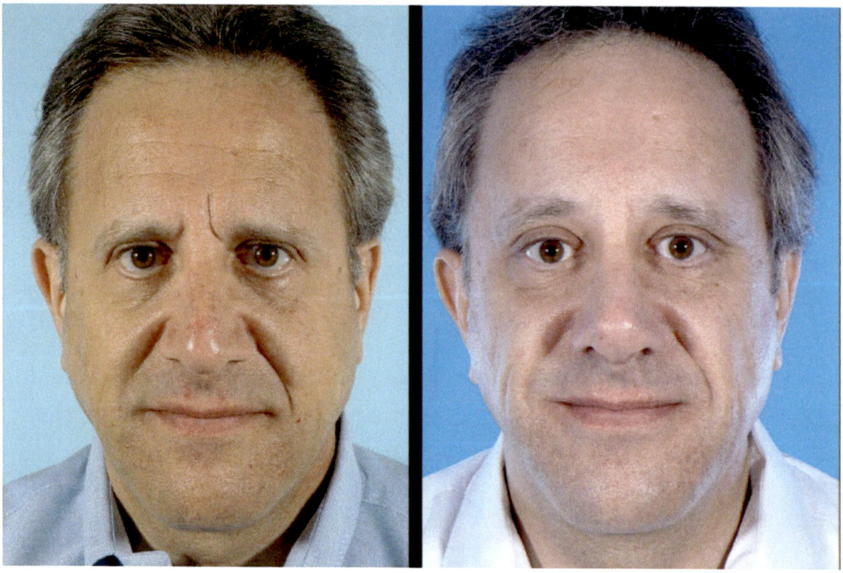

There is still a role for the coronal forehead lift. Besides the forehead lift and correction of the glabellar wrinkling a lateral canthopexy was performed which corrected his scleral show from a previous lower lid blepharopexy. His anterior hairline has been raised, and it could have been shortened with a prefollicular incision and advancement of the frontal hairline.

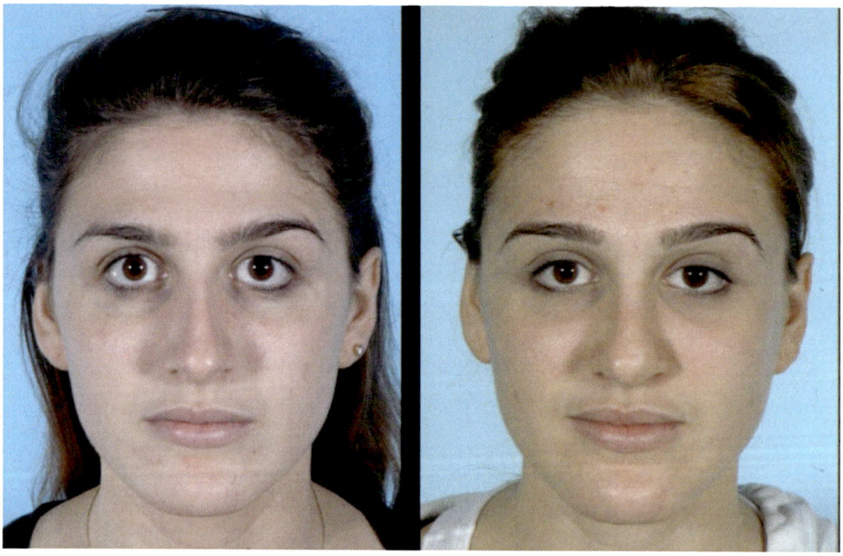

Young woman who felt she looked "sad." Lateral canthopexy and burring of lateral orbital rim performed through coronal incision with forehead lift.

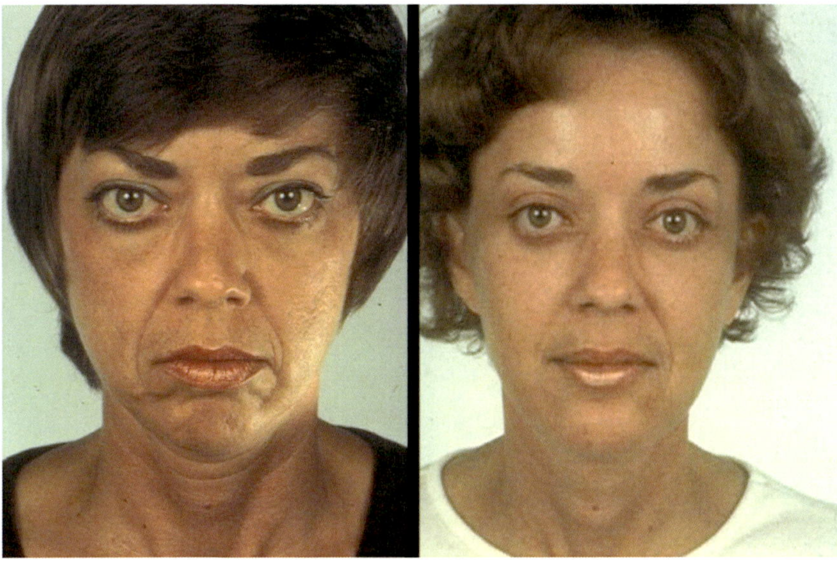

Patient with moderate proptosis from quiescent Grave's disease treated with three wall orbital expansion, genioplasty, and facelift. One should avoid doing a lower lid blepharoplasty without prior expansion of the orbit, since the eyelid will slide under the globe in spite of a good lateral canthopexy.

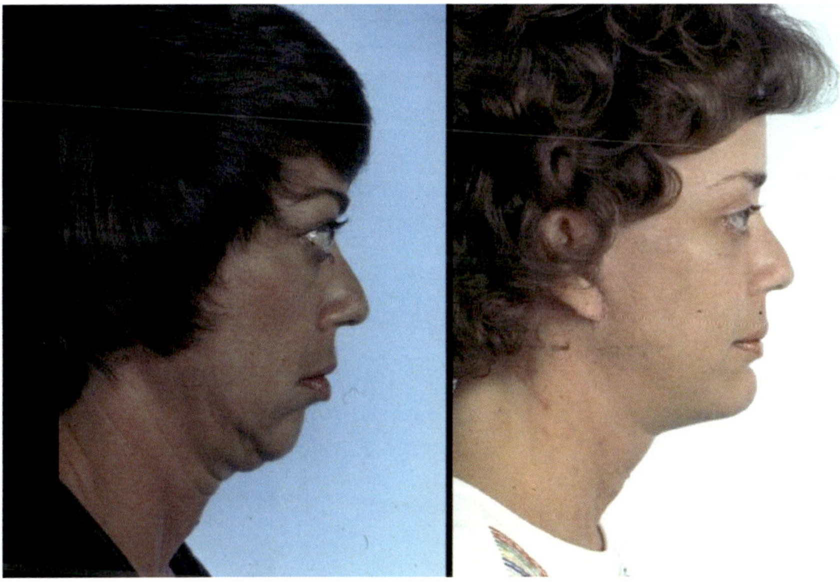

Note posterior movement of globe relative to nasal dorsum.

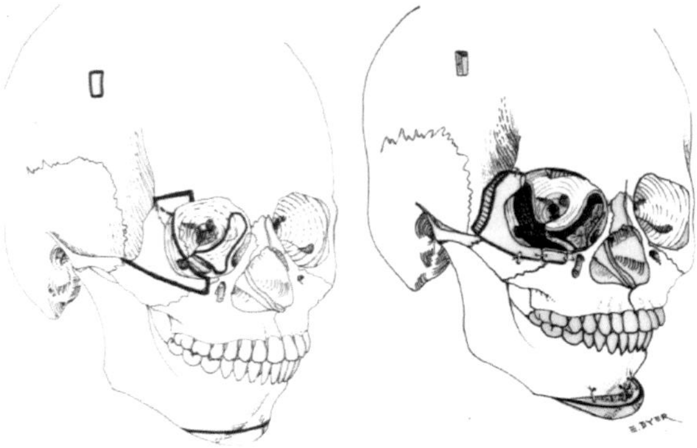

Tessier's original description showed horizontal osteotomy continuing below the zygomatic arch; we carried it above so that there could be an anterior movement of the lateral orbital rim.

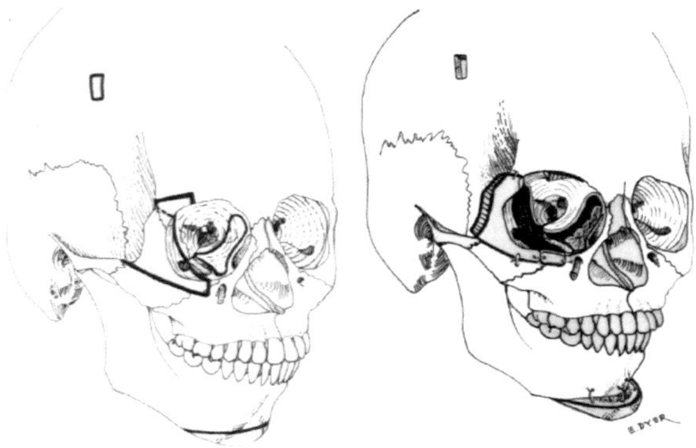

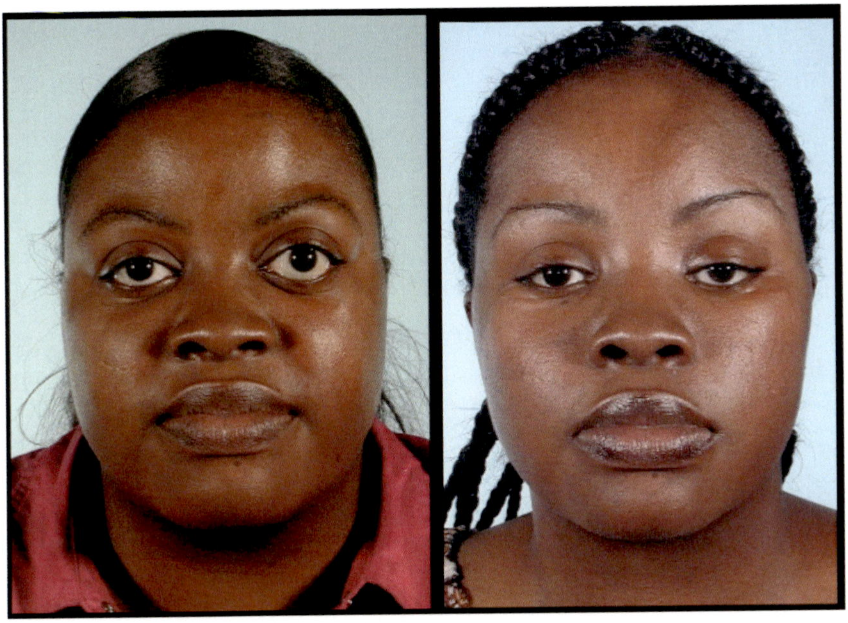

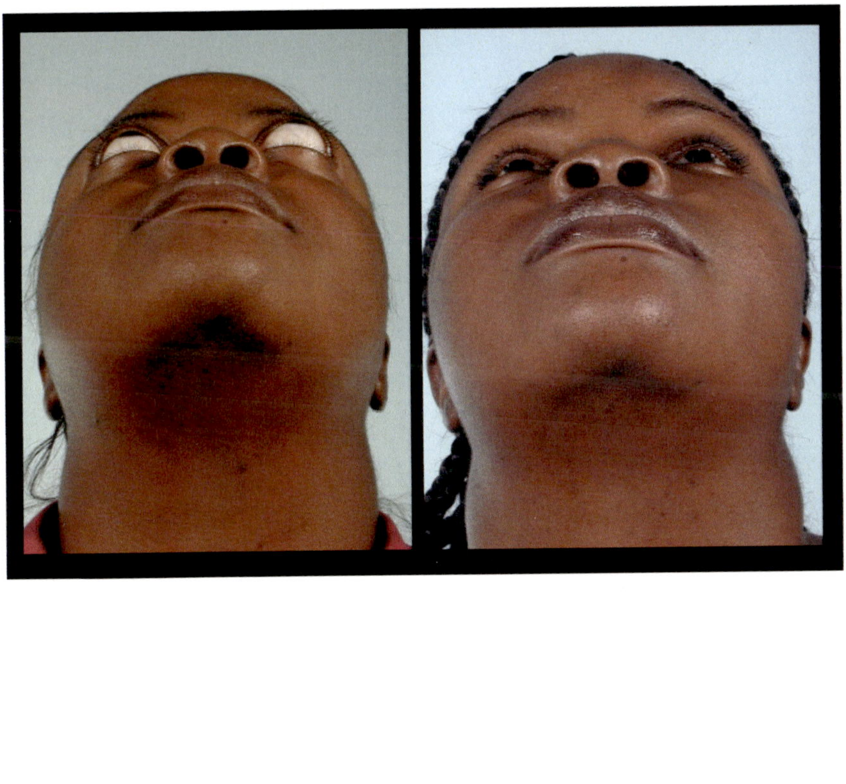

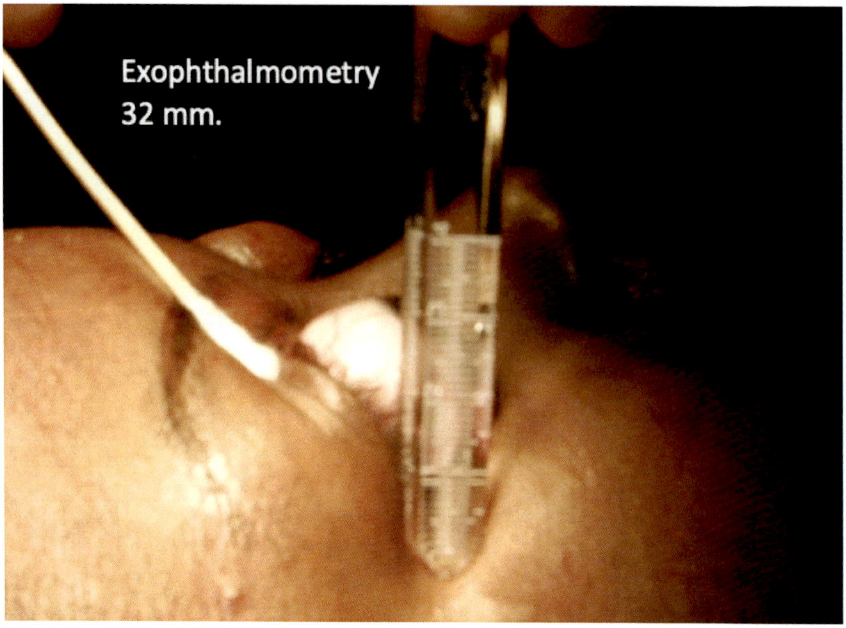

The reading on the left was 34 mm, normal is 16 to 18. These extreme degrees of exophthalmos require as much expansion as possible as well as intraconal fat removal.

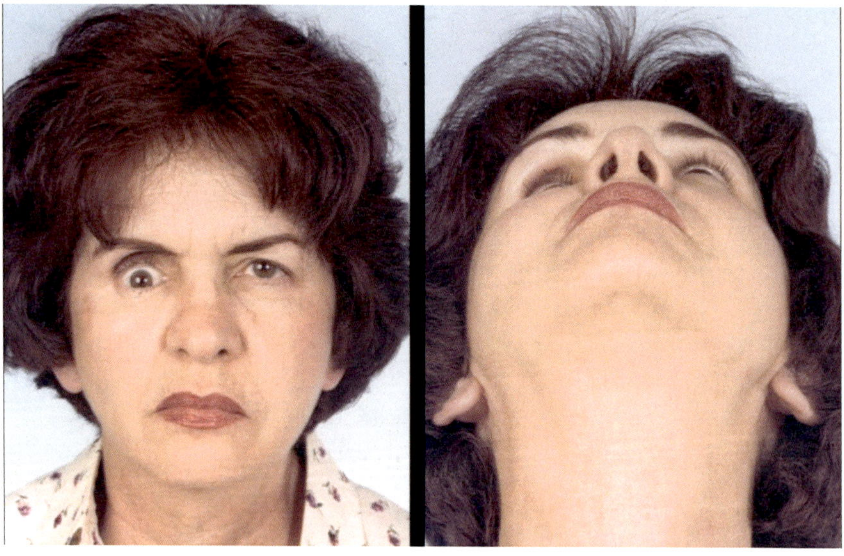

Post-traumatic enophthalmos. CT scan showed a 12 mm difference between anterior surface of corneas. Treated with iliac bone graft for orbital floor and medial wall defects.

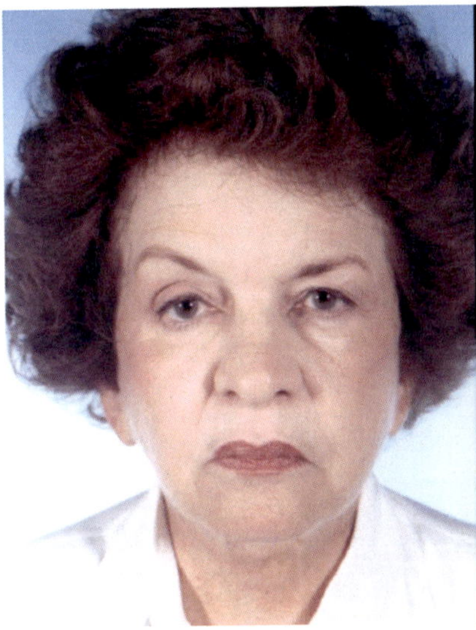

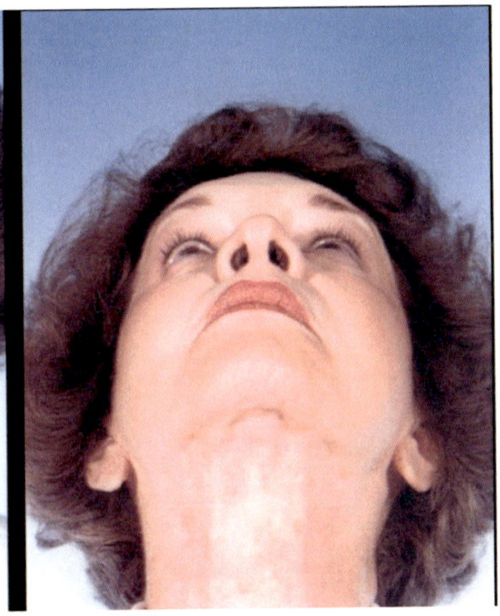

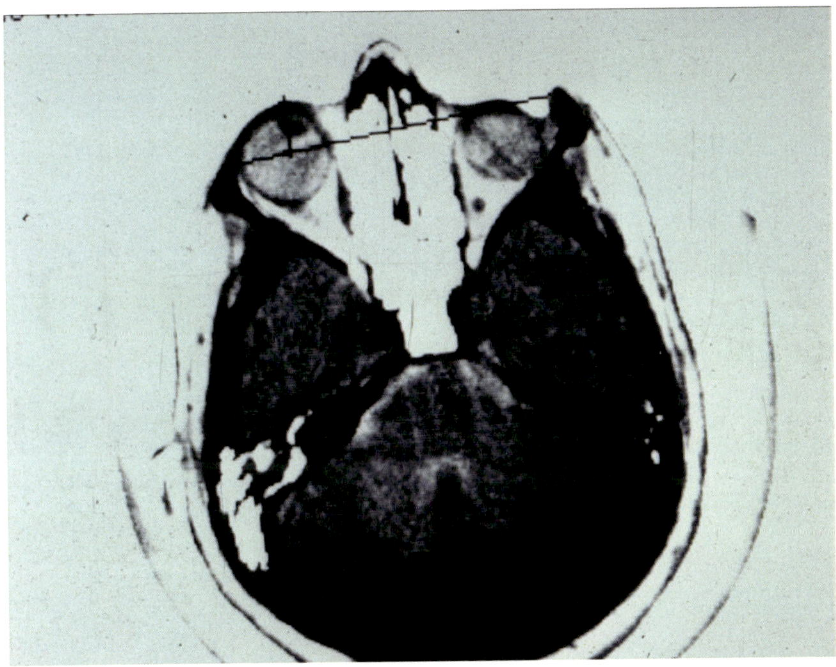

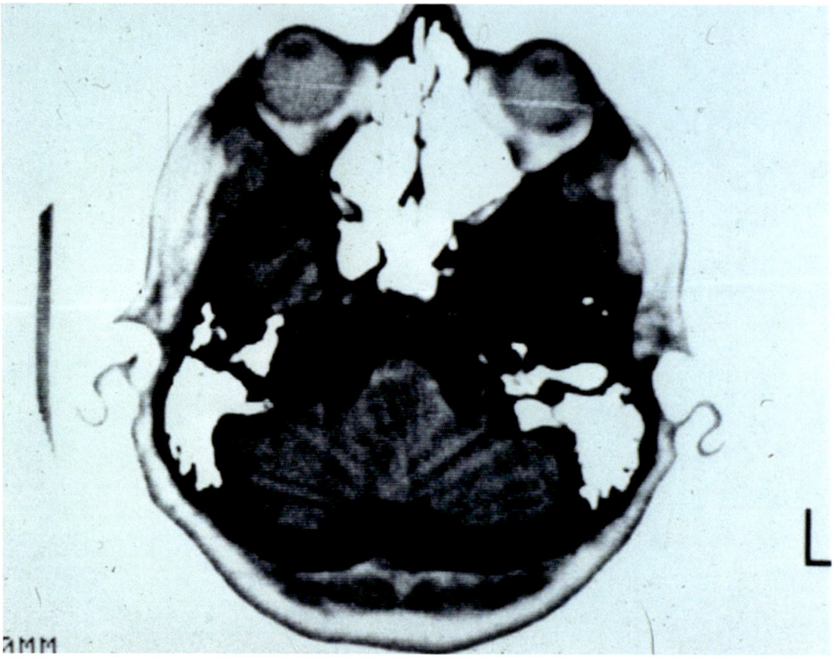

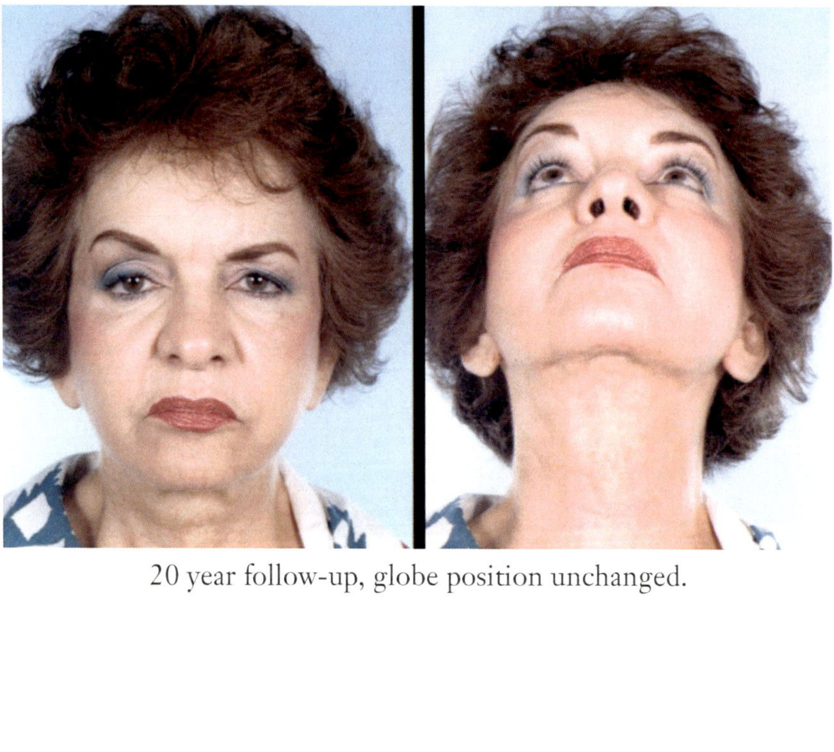

20 year follow-up, globe position unchanged.

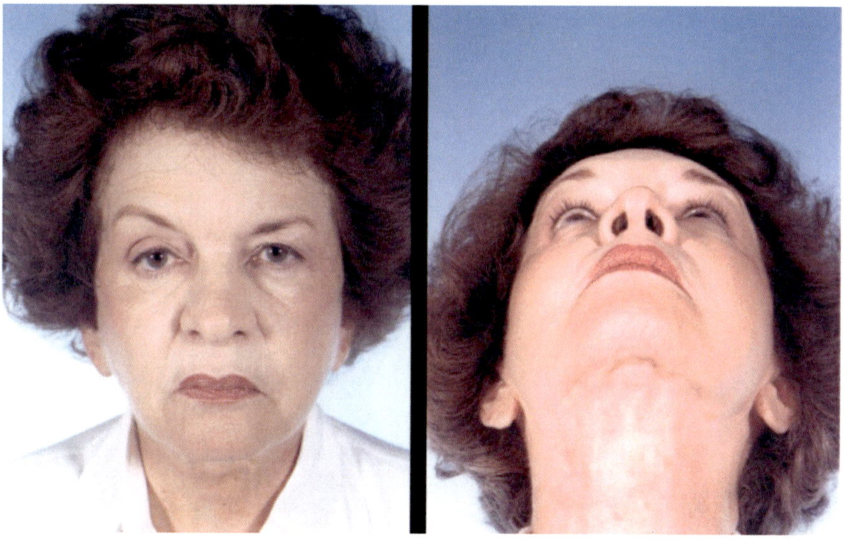

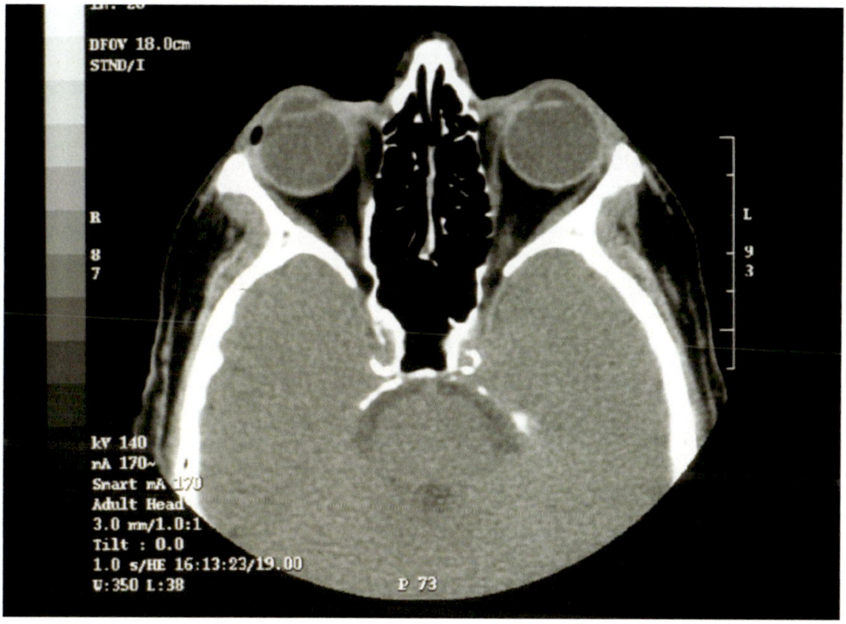

DFOV 18.0cm
STND/I
R
8
7
L
9
3
kV 140
mA 170~
Smart mA 170
Adult Head
3.0 mm/1.0:1
Tilt : 0.0
1.0 s/HE 16:13:23/19.00
W:350 L:38
P 73

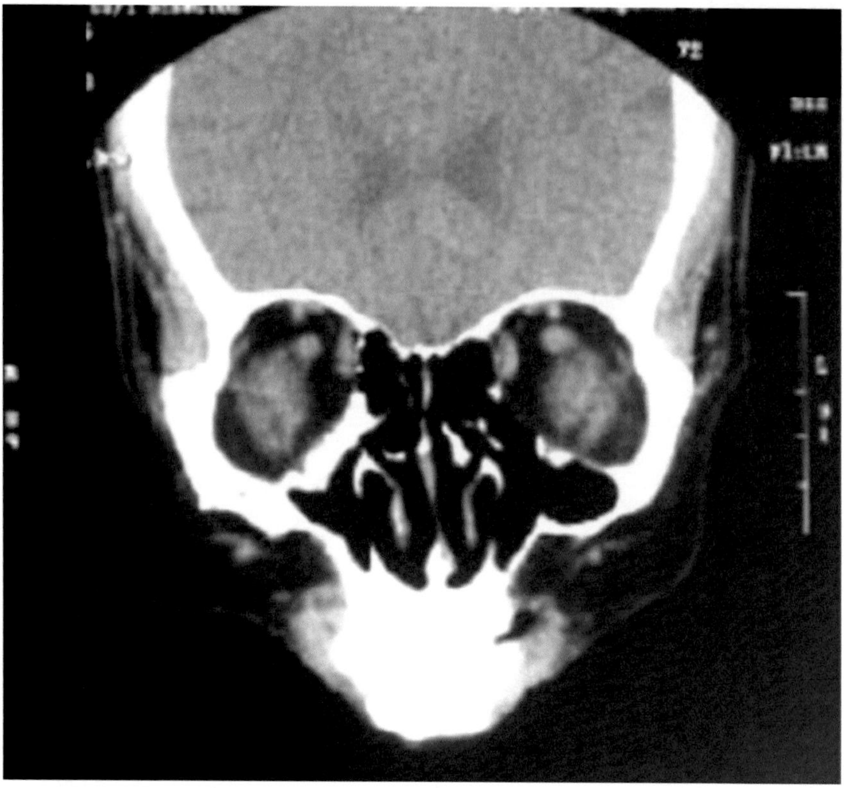

The thicker orbital floor on the right is the iliac bone graft after 20 years.

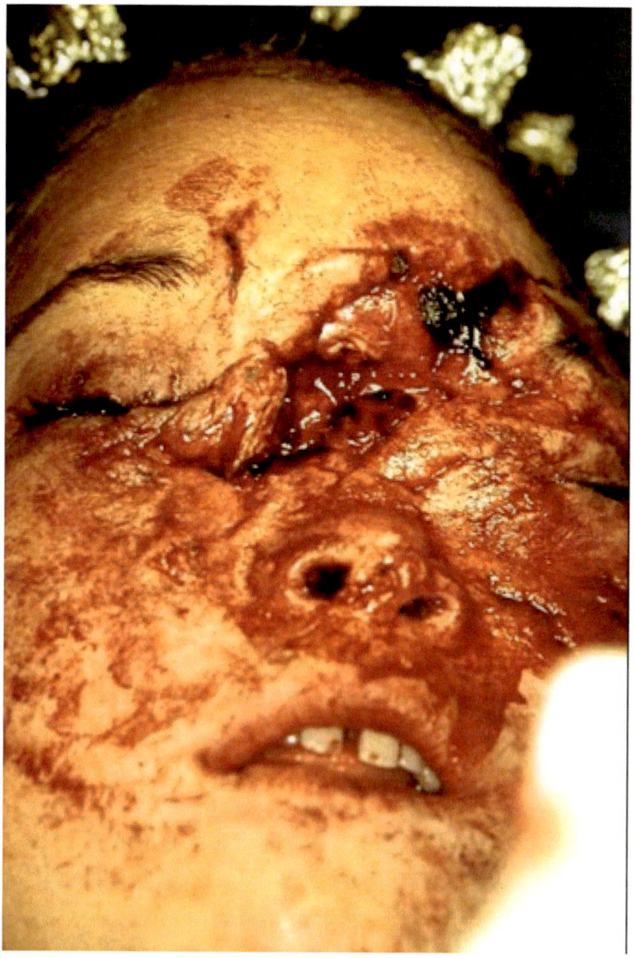

Automobile accident. Left globe ruptured. Similar to case shown earlier from residency, but with greater soft tissue injury in interorbital area. Diastema of maxilla evident. indicating midline maxillary fracture.

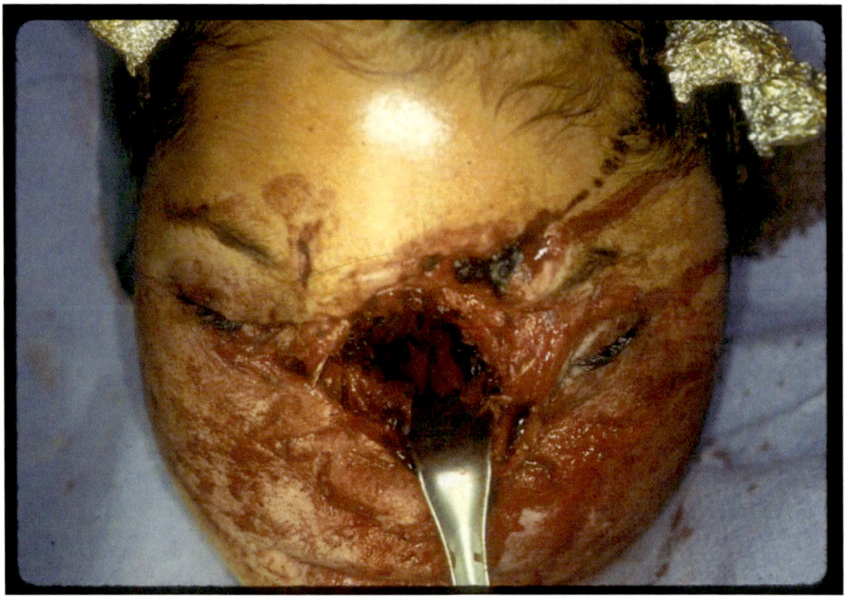

View of pharynx.

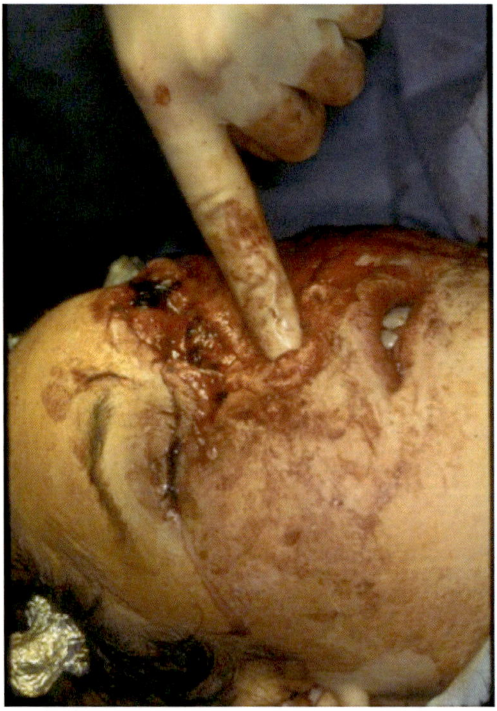

Positive "Gruss sign" wherein nose can be pushed to pharynx.

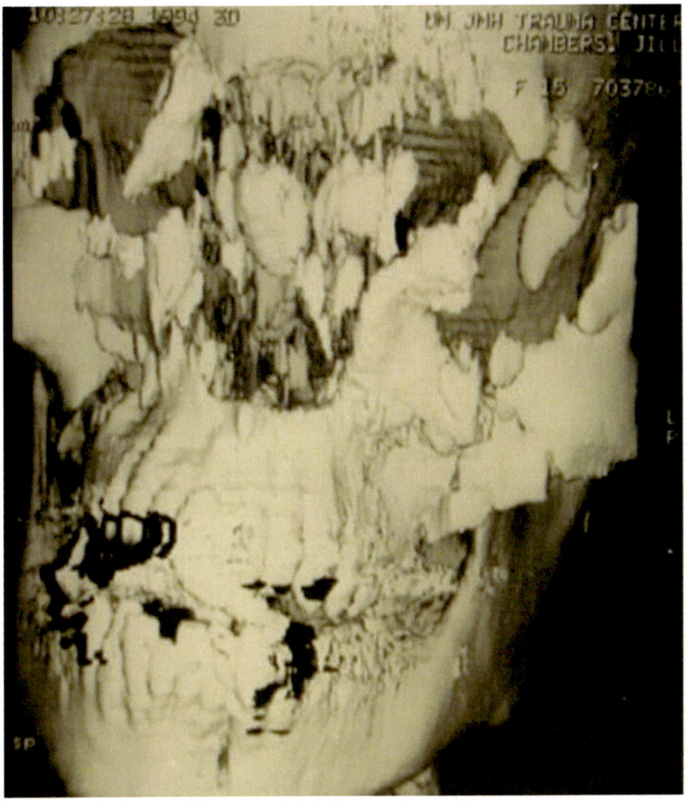

This is truly a “pan-facial” fracture, bilateral orbitozygomatic, naso-orbital ethmoid, maxillary, mandibular, left condylar dislocation. The case is similar to Richard L———, the one I did as a resident before exposure to Tessier, but worse due to the nasal fractures and nasal soft tissue damage requiring an eventual forehead flap. Were I to do it again, I would further lengthen the nose. Except for the forehead flap, everything was corrected at the primary operation, with large amounts of calvarial and iliac bone grafts.

A second forehead flap might be considered.

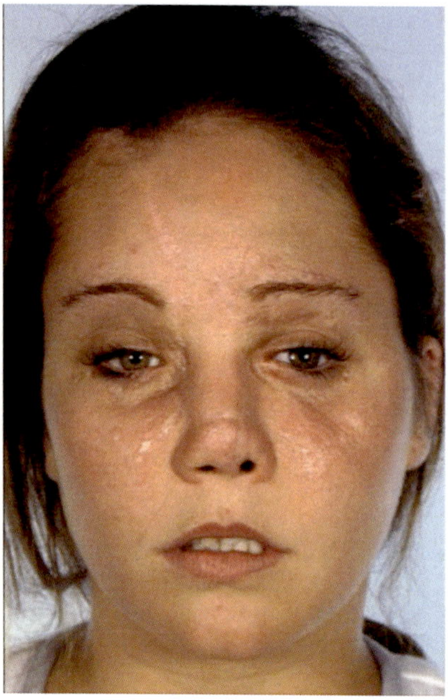

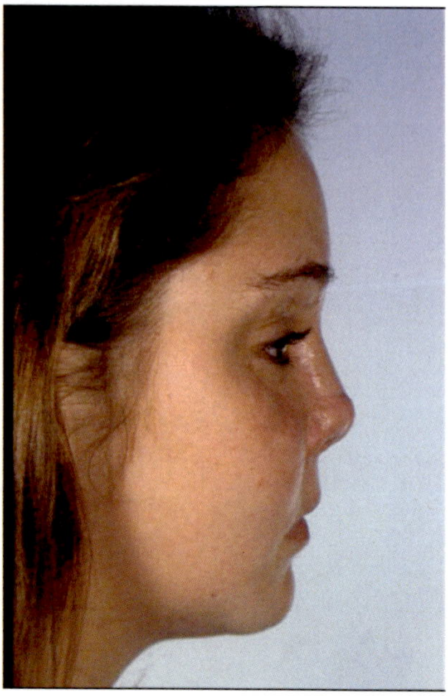

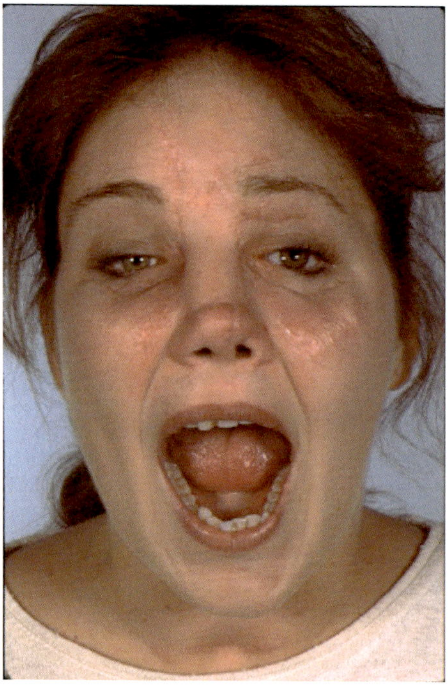

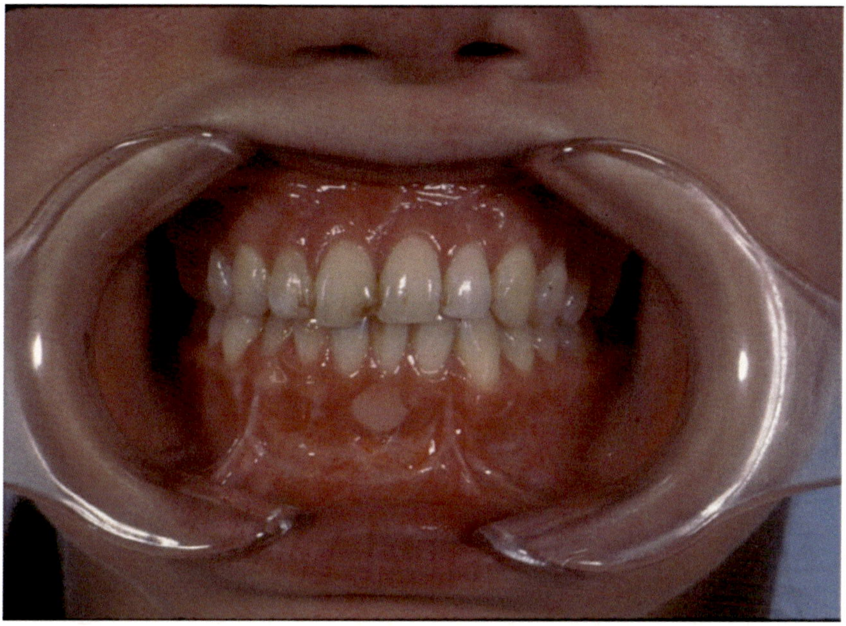

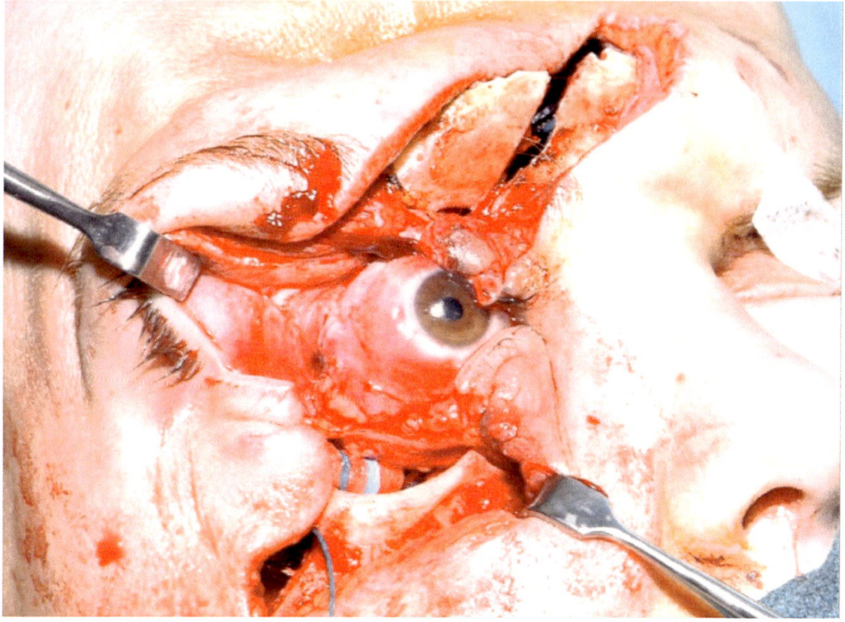

Propeller injury from having a boat back over her in Biscayne Bay. Kerf of blade evident in medial orbit and glabella. Globe somehow spared.

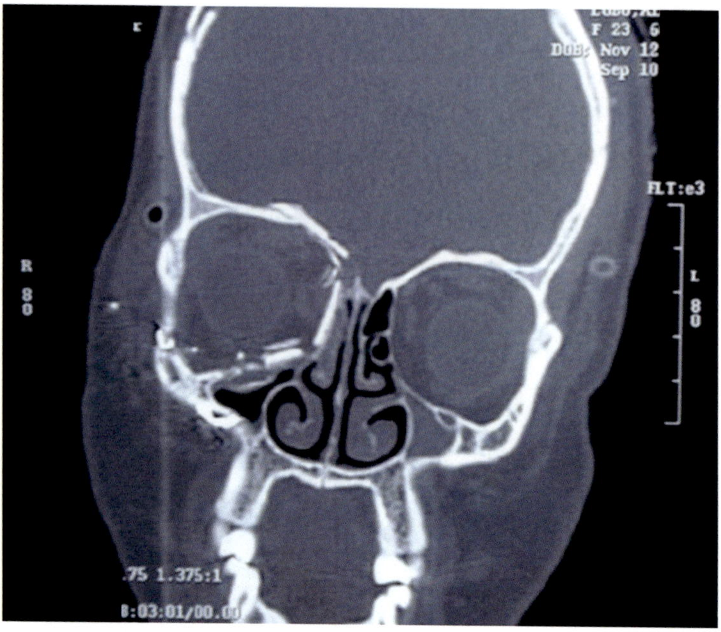

Primary calvarial bone grafts to medial orbital wall, orbital floor, anterior maxilla, and orbital roof.

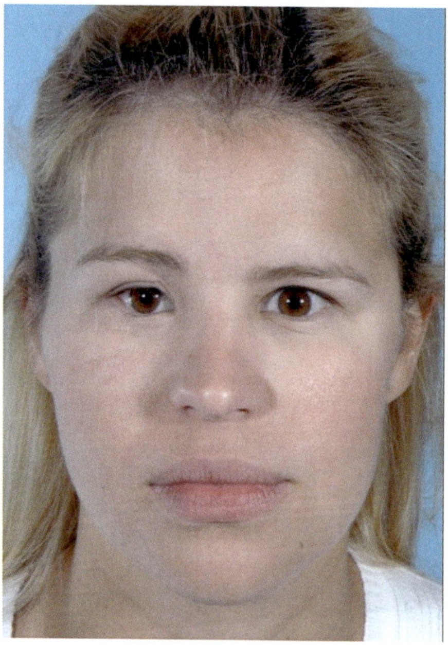

Five-year follow up with one secondary procedure to add a bit more bone across inferior orbital fissure to correct 2 mm of enophthalmos.

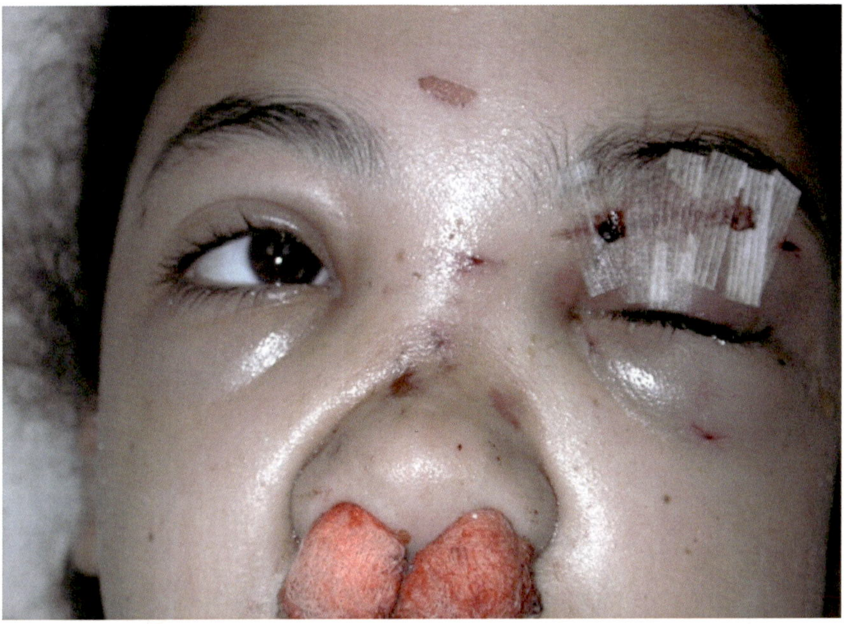

Unrestrained back seat passenger flew over seat to hit dashboard. Telecanthus is evident. Nasal collapse.

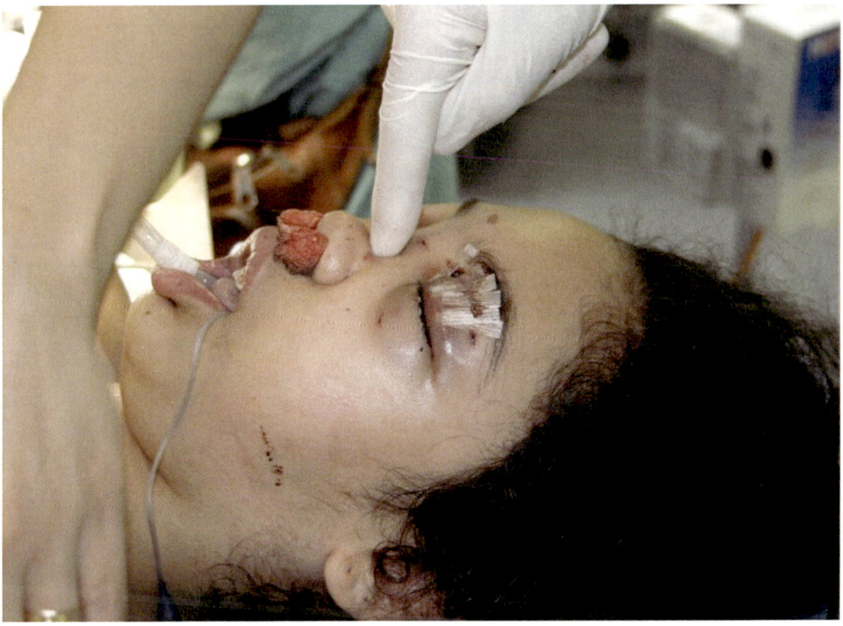

Another positive Gruss sign.

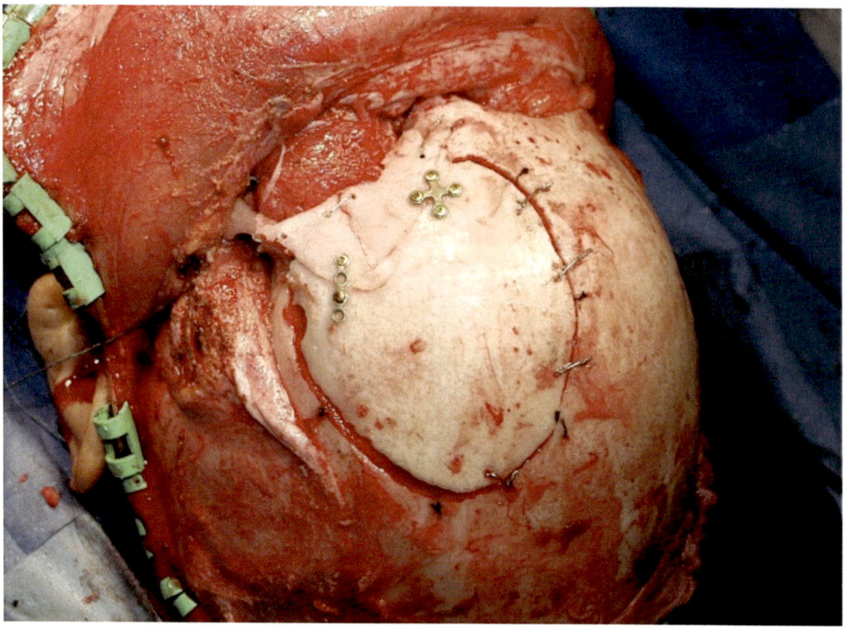

The neurosurgeons did a frontal craniotomy to close a dural tear, more than enough bone for nasal and bilateral orbital floor bone grafts could be harvested from inner table of their cranial bone flap.

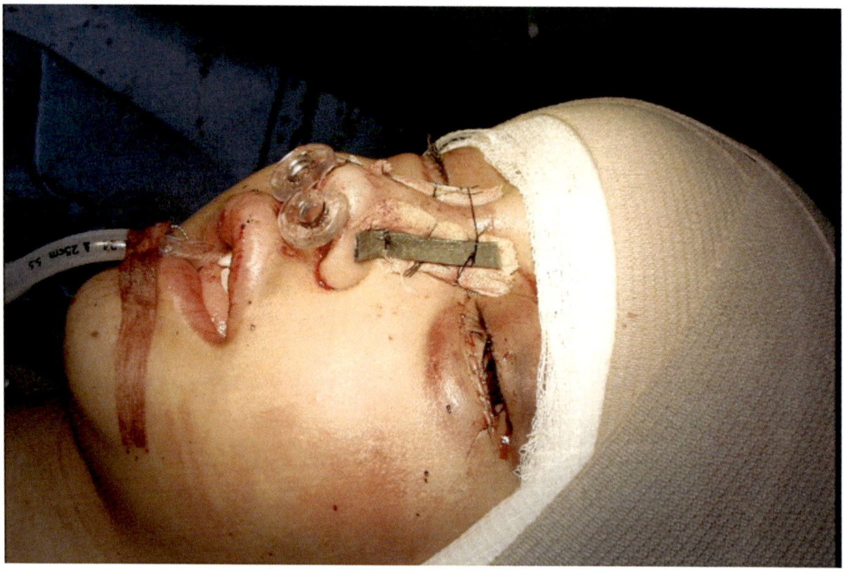

Besides a nasal bone graft, a conchal cartilage graft was placed in the nasal tip. Reduction and rigid fixation of medial orbital wall and medial canthi and orbitozygomatic fracture carried out through subtarsal lower incisions.

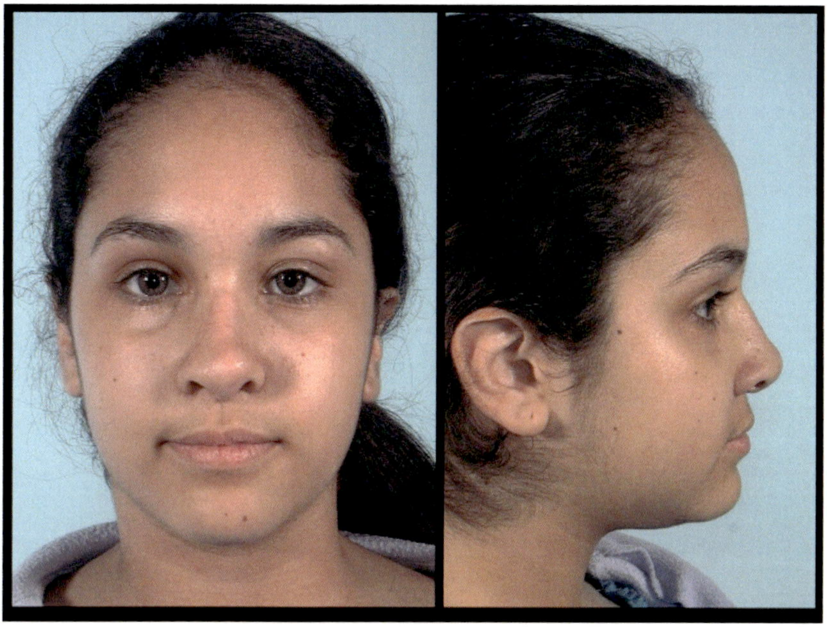

Six-month result with no further surgery. Slight retraction of columellar base incision evident.

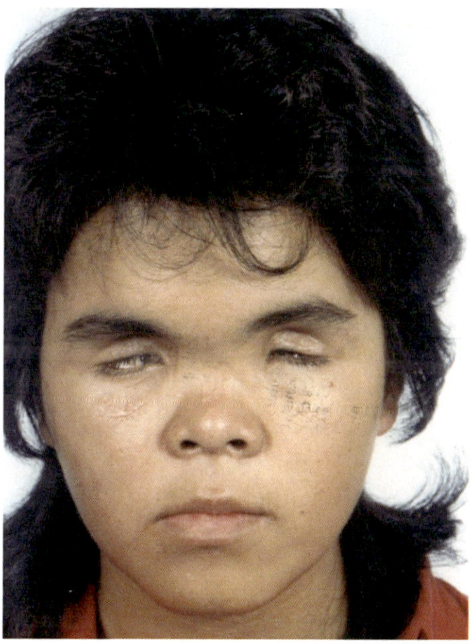

Fifteen-year-old girl involved in auto accident in Bolivia. Lost vision both eyes. Nasoorbital ethmoid injury with Le Fort 1 fracture. Class 3 malocclusion. Treatment was extensive dissection to release scarring followed by nasal bone graft, Le Fort 1 osteotomy and advancement, medial canthopexies. Shown at 25 years post op with no further surgery.

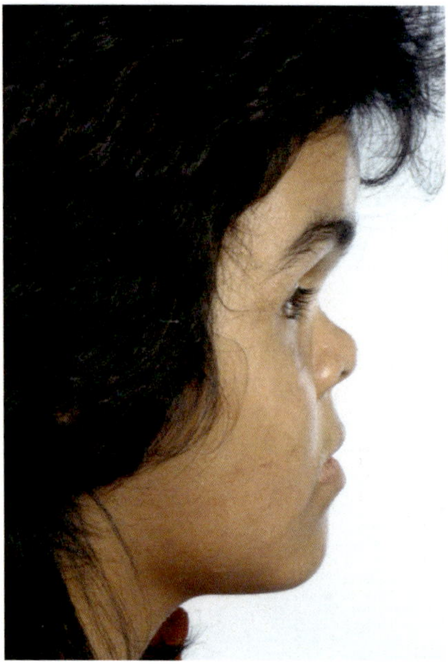

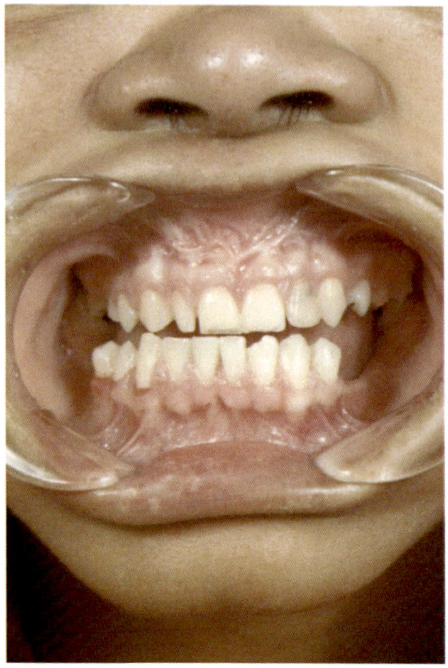

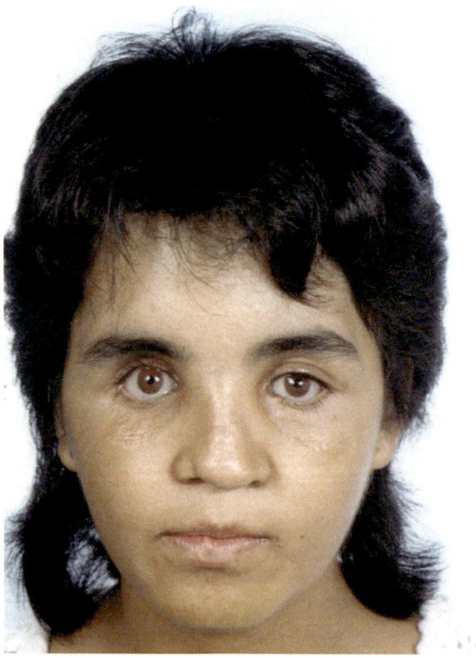

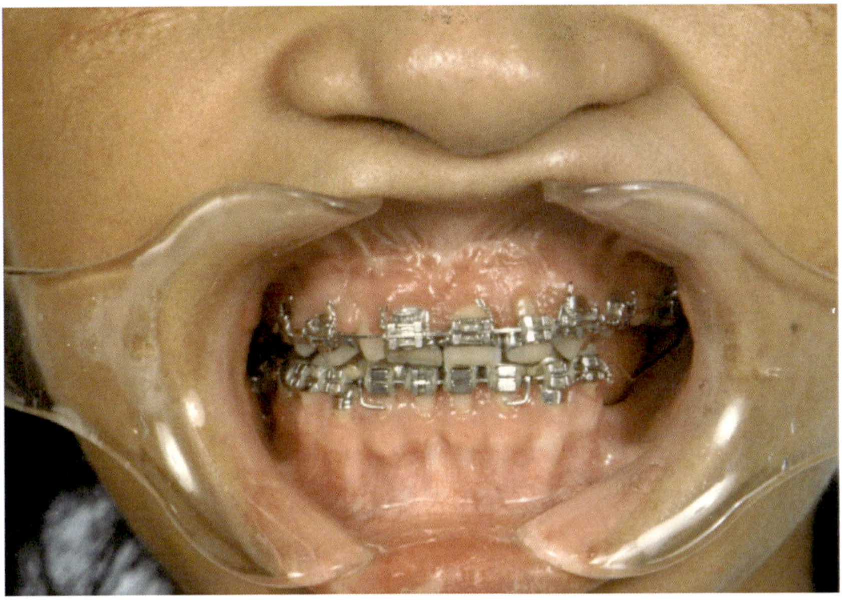

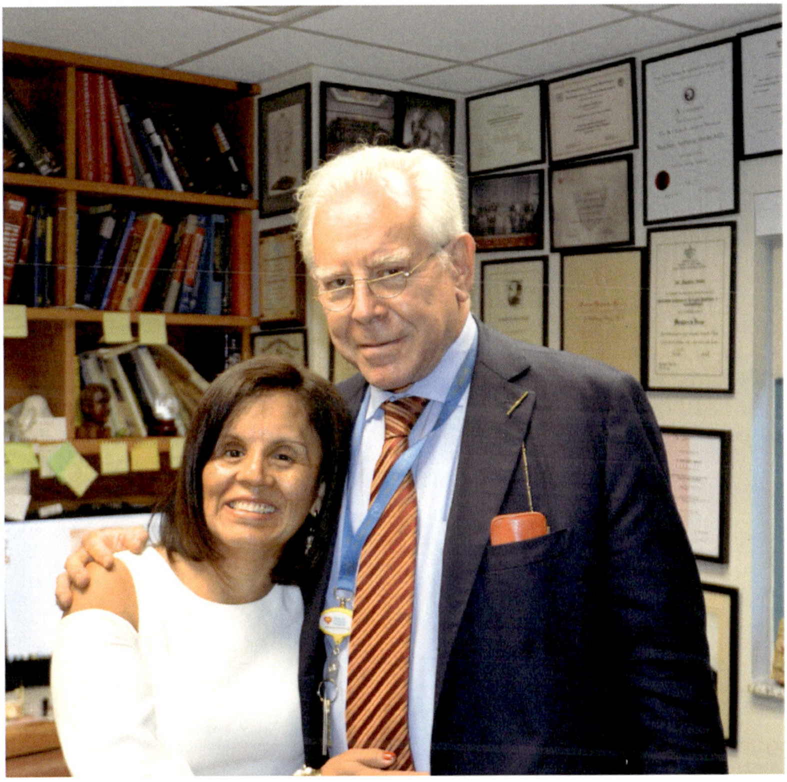

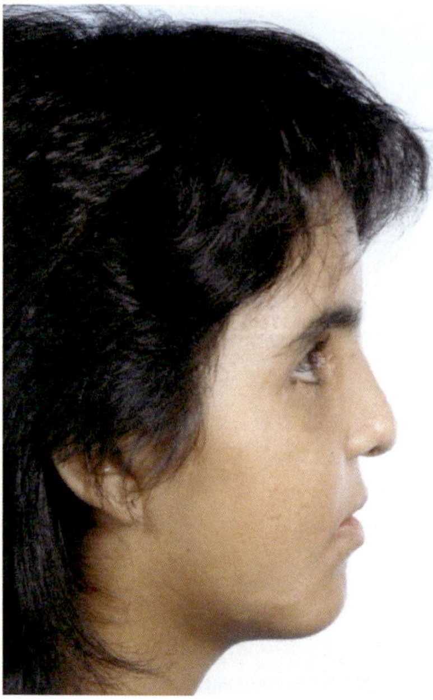

Twenty-five year followup. Occlusion good, no resorption of nasal bone graft.

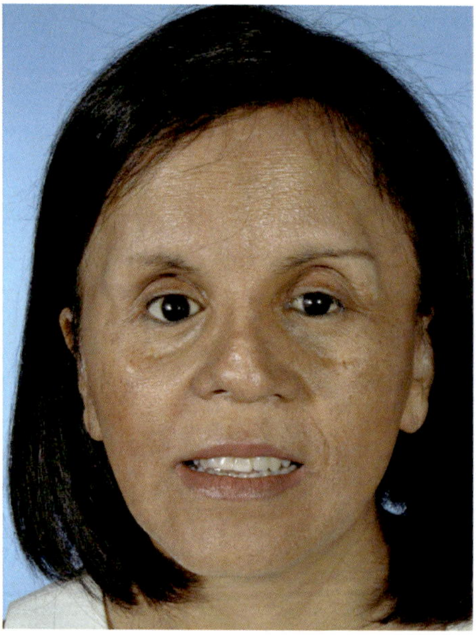

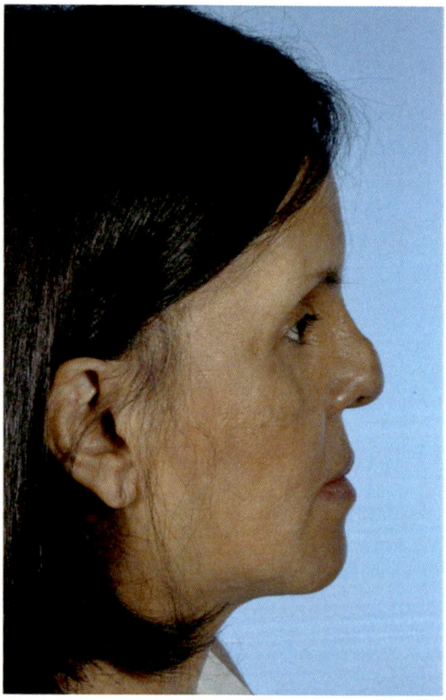

Twenty-five-year followup. There has been no resorption of the nasal bone graft, in fact, there has been some accretional growth in the supratip area which was treated by burring it down and some lipofilling of the periorbital areas (shown 2 days post op).

First vertical, then horizontal.

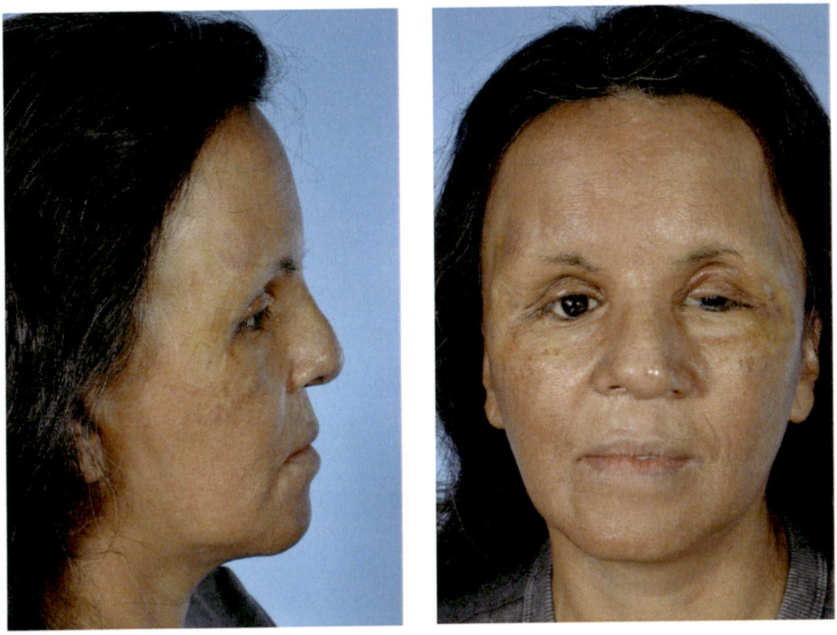

Vertical orbital dystopia

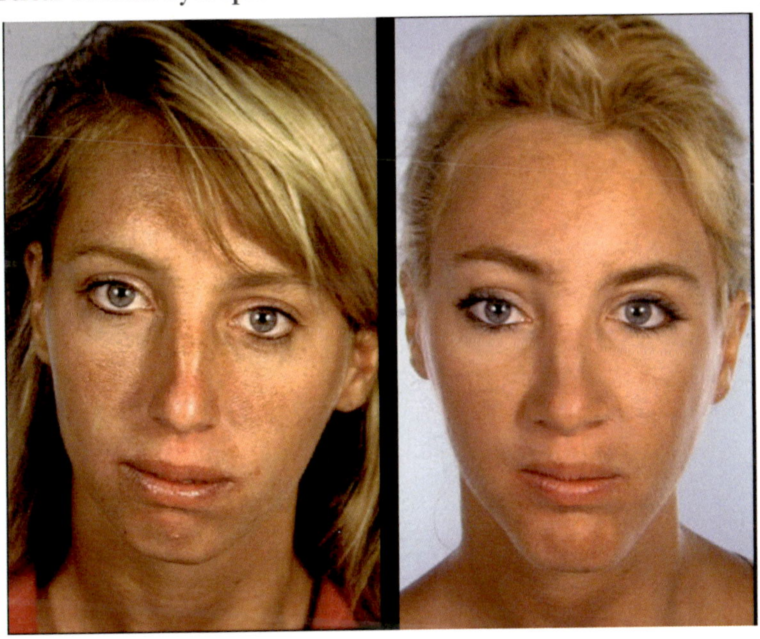

Pronounced facial asymmetry due to left tortcolllis.

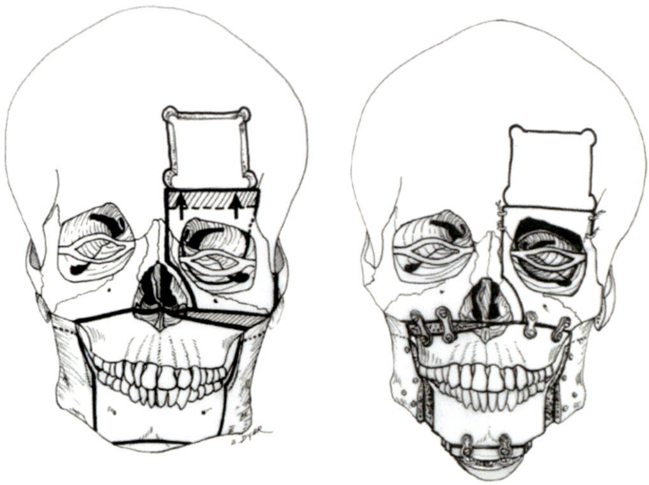

One stage procedure with correction of vertical orbital dystopia and maxillomandibular distortion, with lengthening genioplasty.

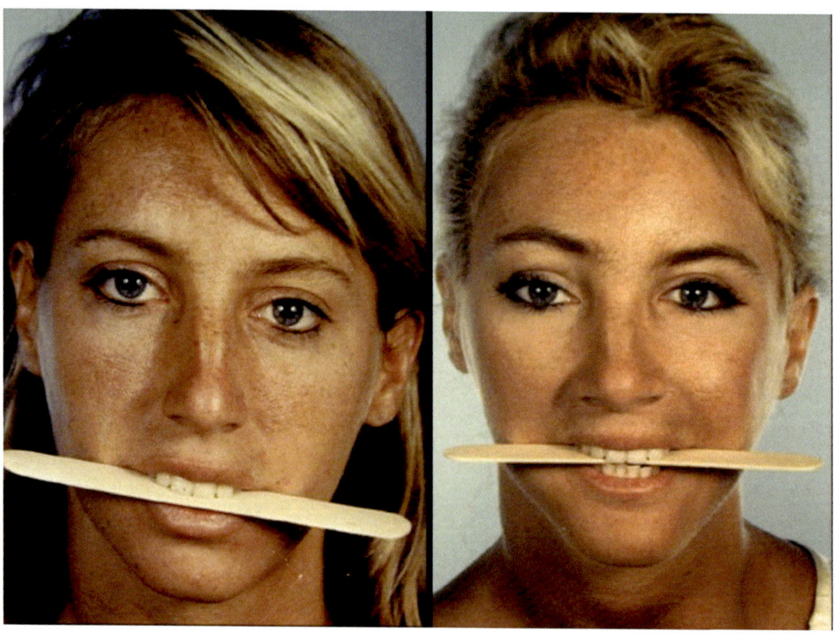

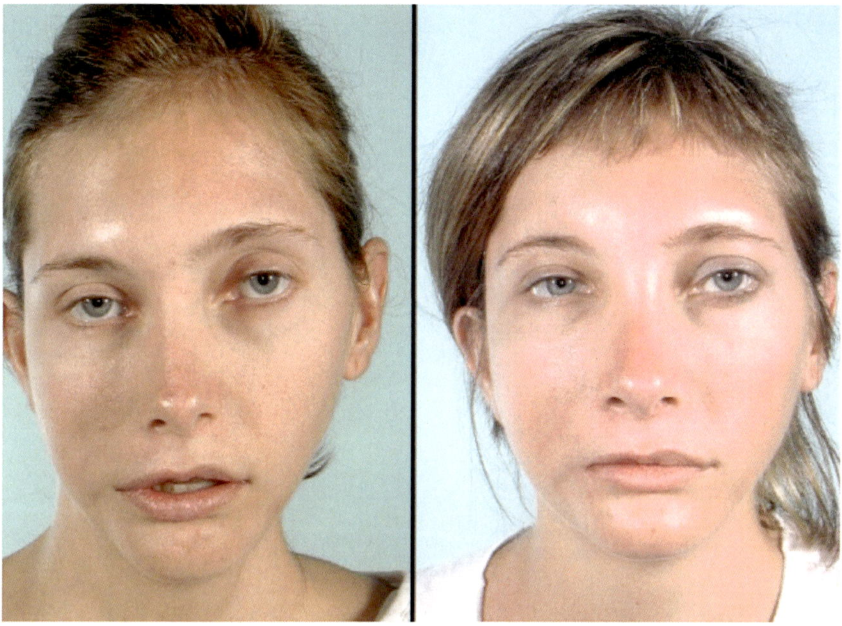

Another orbital dystopia due to torticollis. Now using minimally invasive technique. Here only one burr hole was made in the lateral orbit to expose and protect the dura. The rest of the bone strip is removed from the frontal sinus, extracranially. There is no craniotomy flap.

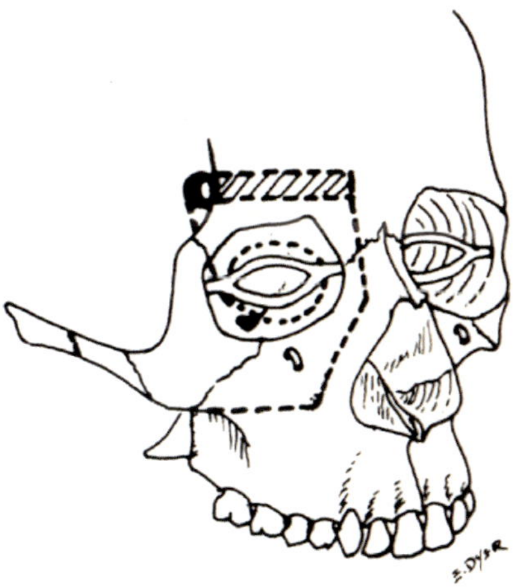

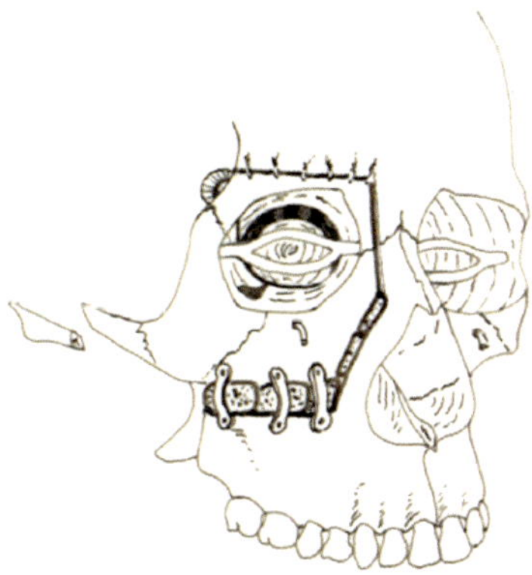

Hypertelorism

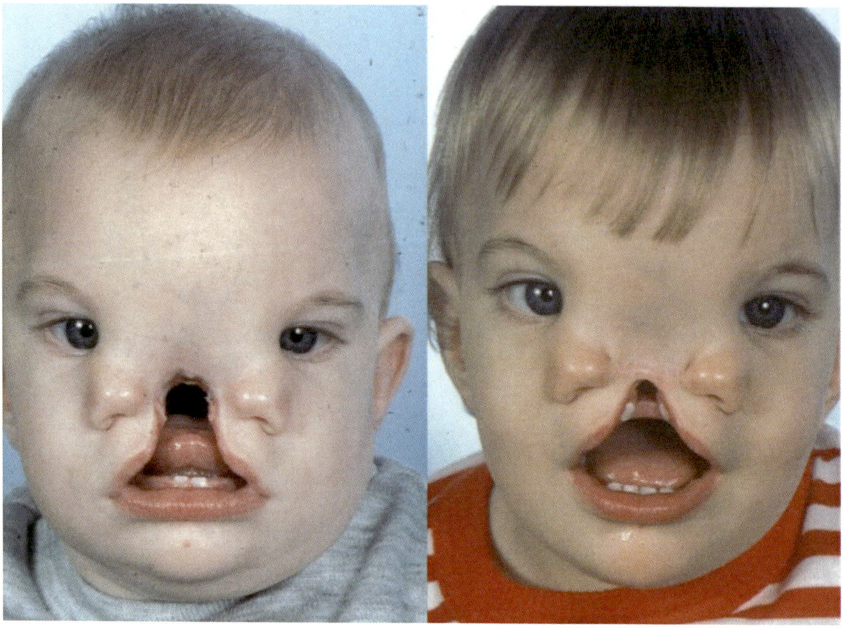

0-14 cleft treated by facial bipartition.

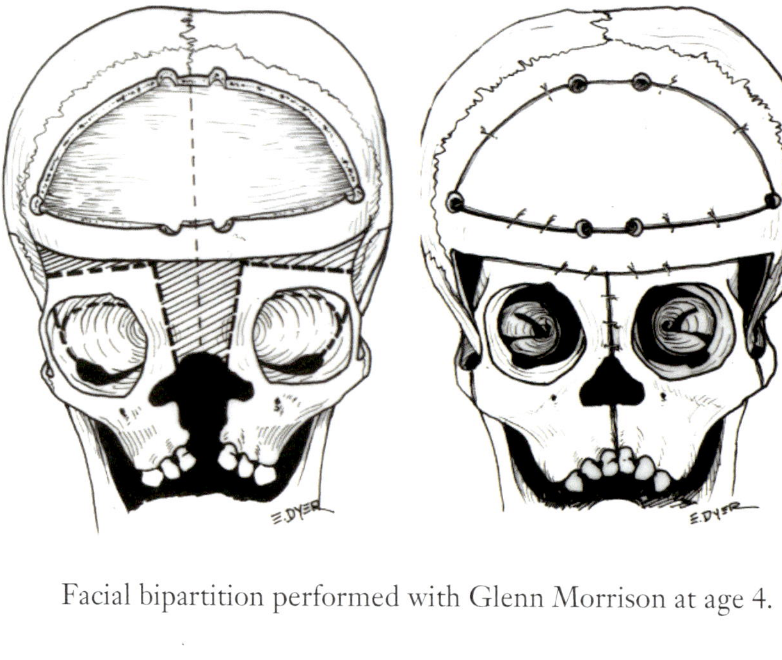

Facial bipartition performed with Glenn Morrison at age 4.

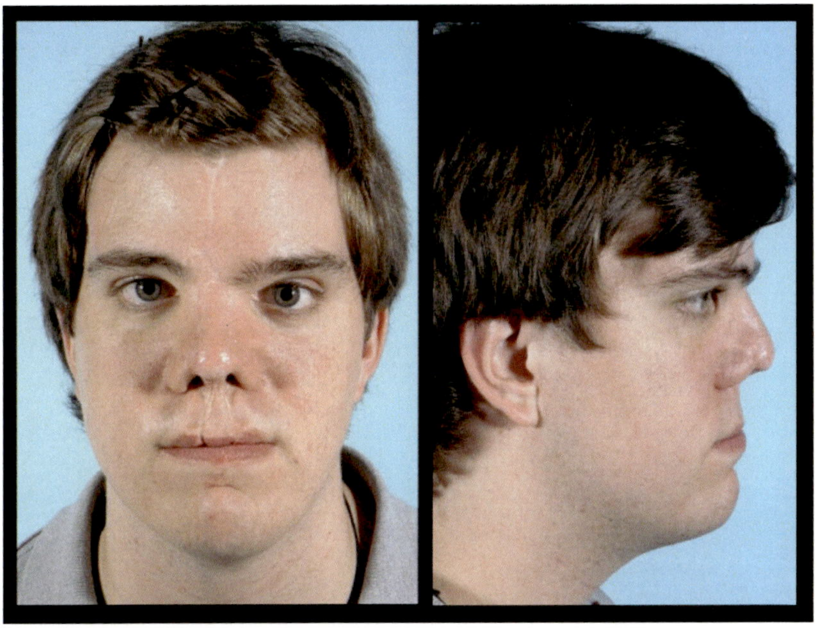

Final result after Le Fort 1 and secondary forehead flap.

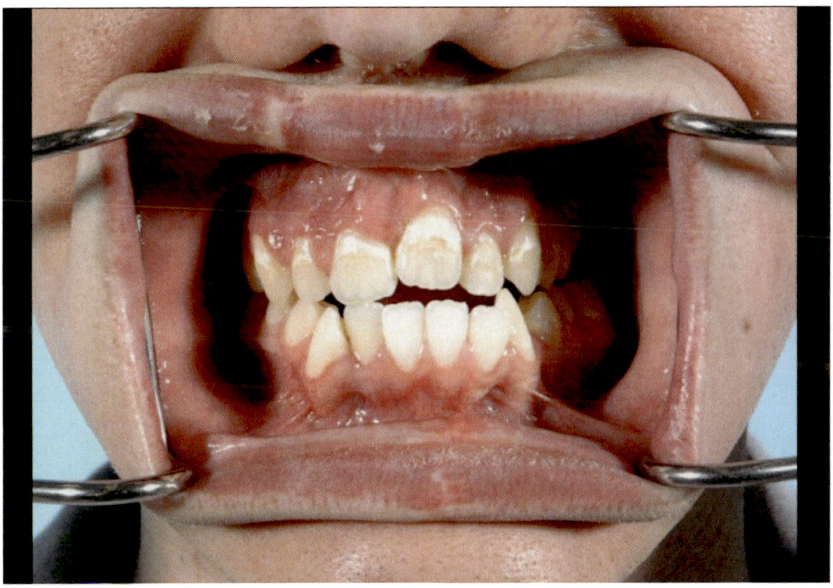

Use of a paramedian forehead flap as a final step in hypertelorism patients brings the eyebrows properly together and trades the midline nasal scar for two dorsal aesthetic lines and can provide tissue for further tip projection, which this patient could have used.

Hypotelorism

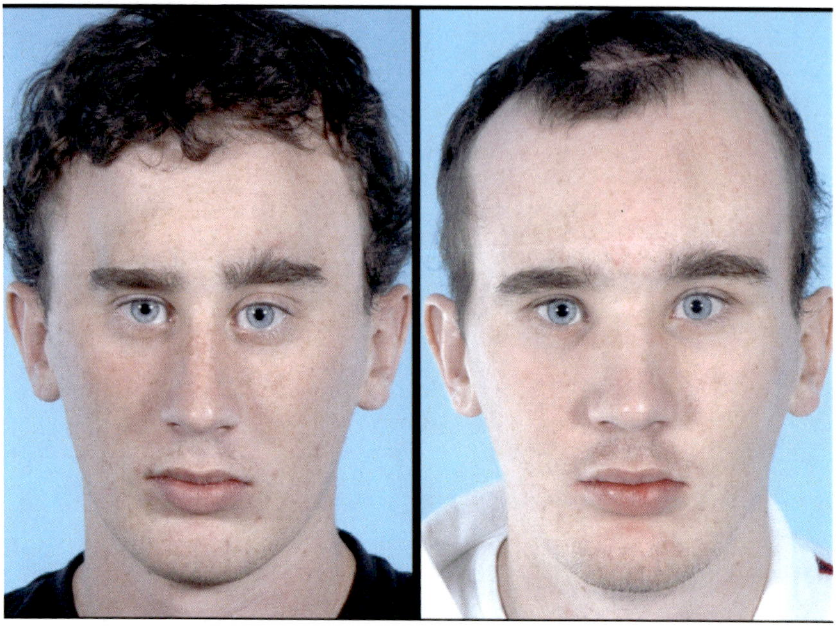

Patient after inadequate trigonocephaly correction. Hypotelorism is easier to correct than hyper, since nothing need be done for the nose.

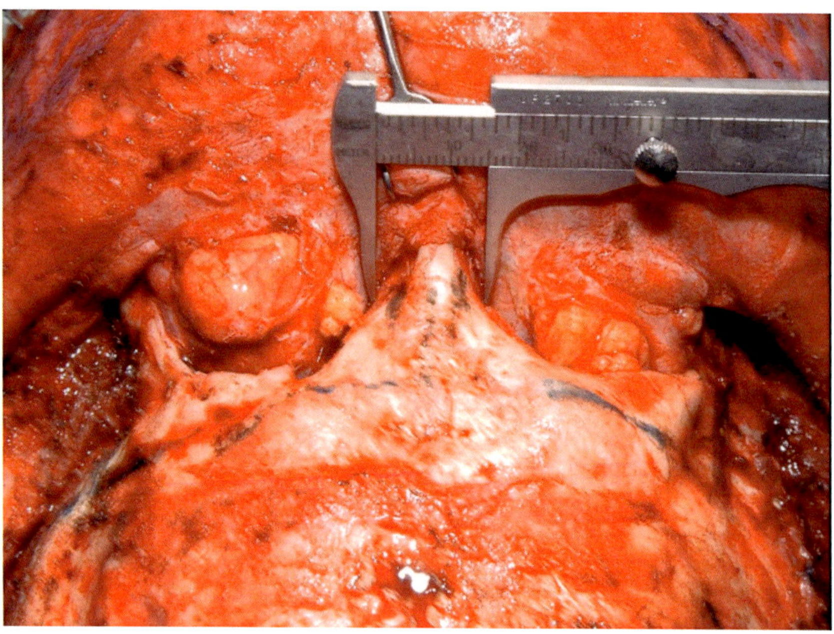

Interorbital distance of 15, which should be 25 or more in an adult.

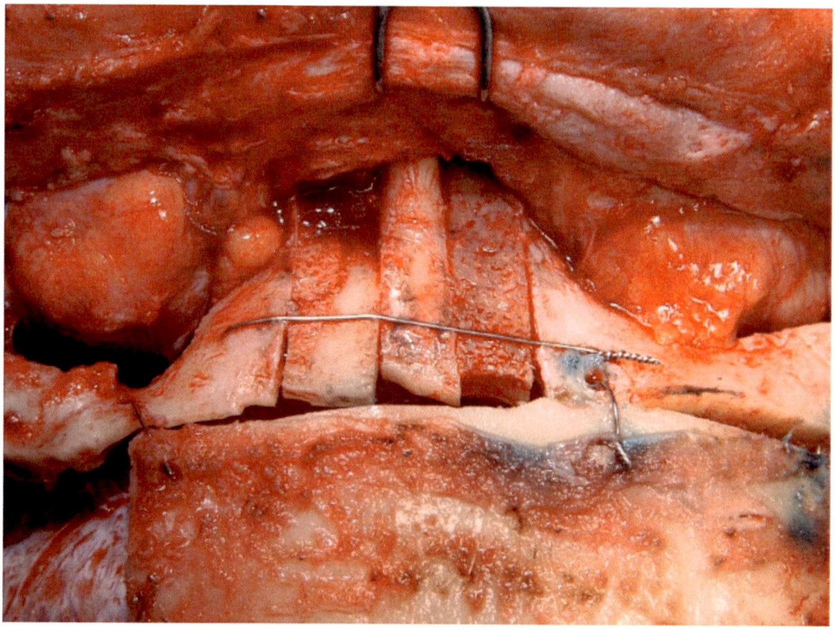

Corrected to 26 mm.

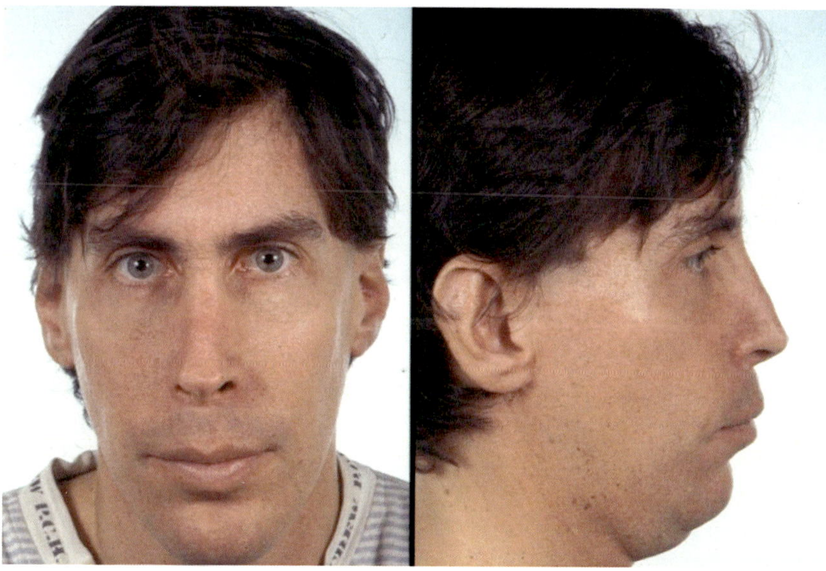

Patient with malar, chin, and nasal implants and significant hypotelorism. The implants were removed and the box osteotomies extended to the malar bones, and both orbito-malar, segments displaced laterally to provide correction of the hypotelorism along with malar augmentation. He also had a genioplasty.

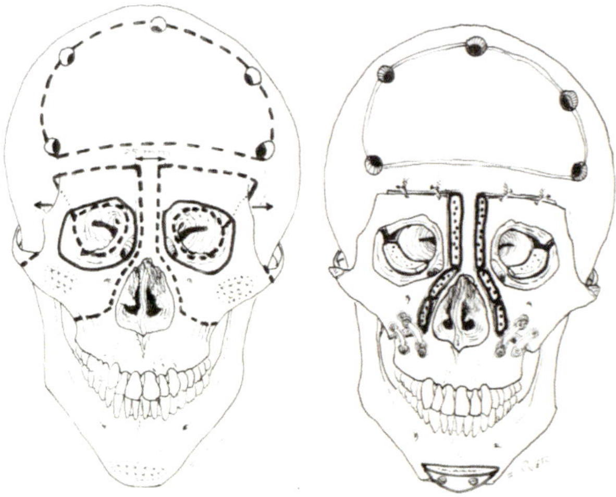

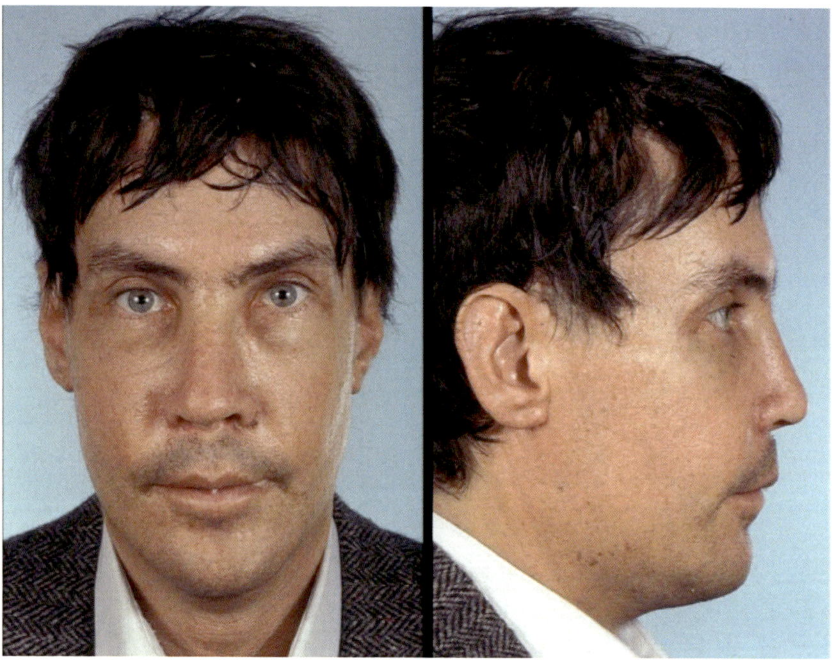

Some might label this patient as having body dysmorphic syndrome, but I don't agree. I would use a different term: facial dysphoria syndrome. This is a condition seen primarily in young men seeking major surgery to alter their face, but unlike body dysmorphic syndrome they are happy with the outcome, but often come back wanting more.

Genioplasty

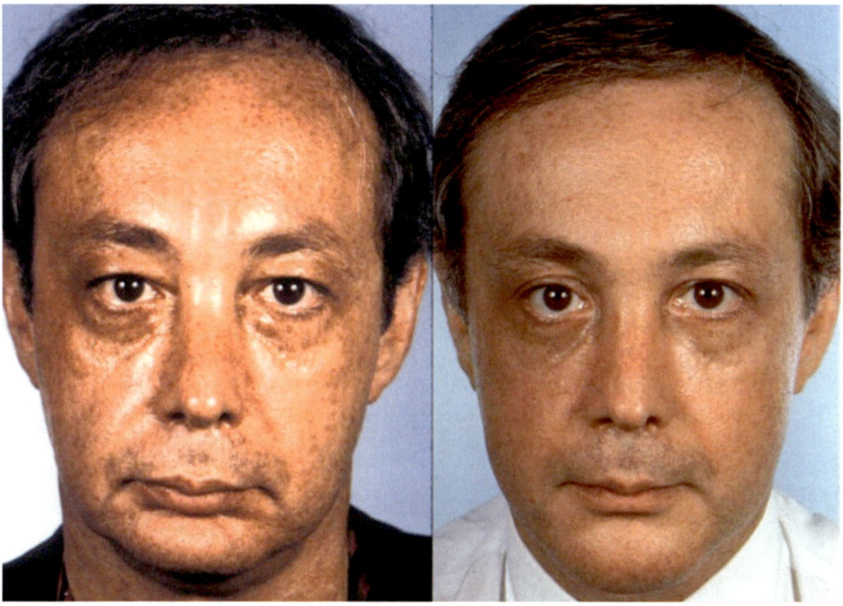

This physician had had a chin implant placed, with an inadequate result due to the shortness of the chin. The implant was removed, and the chin lengthened with an interpositional bone graft. Also face lift and blepharoplasties.

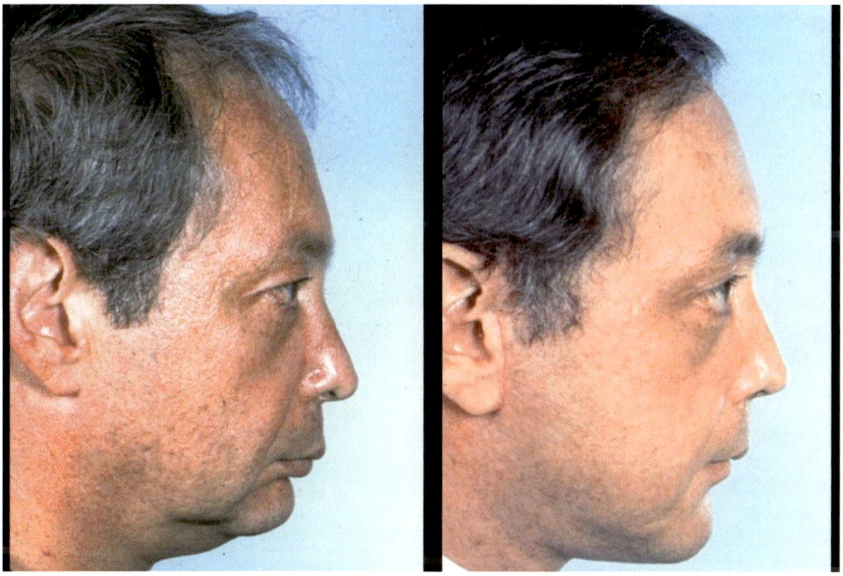

Note the effacement of the labiomental crease, like the opening of an accordion.

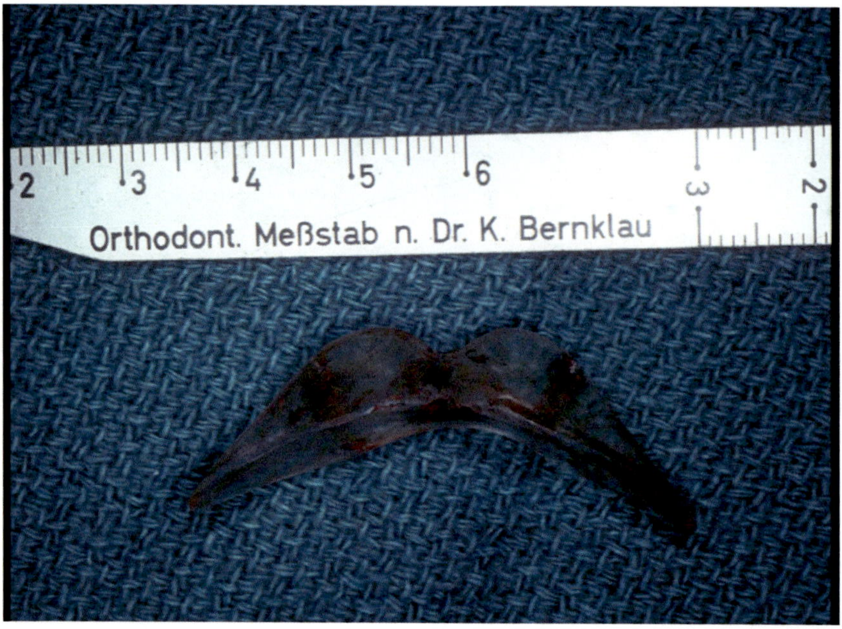
2 3 4 5 6
Orthodont. Meßstab n. Dr. K. Bernklau

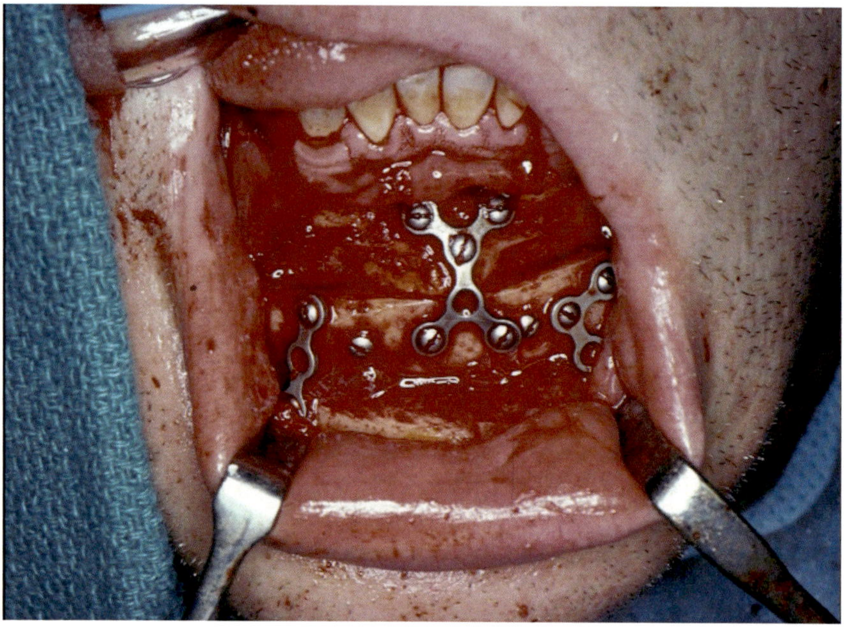

Staged genioplasties for maximal effect.

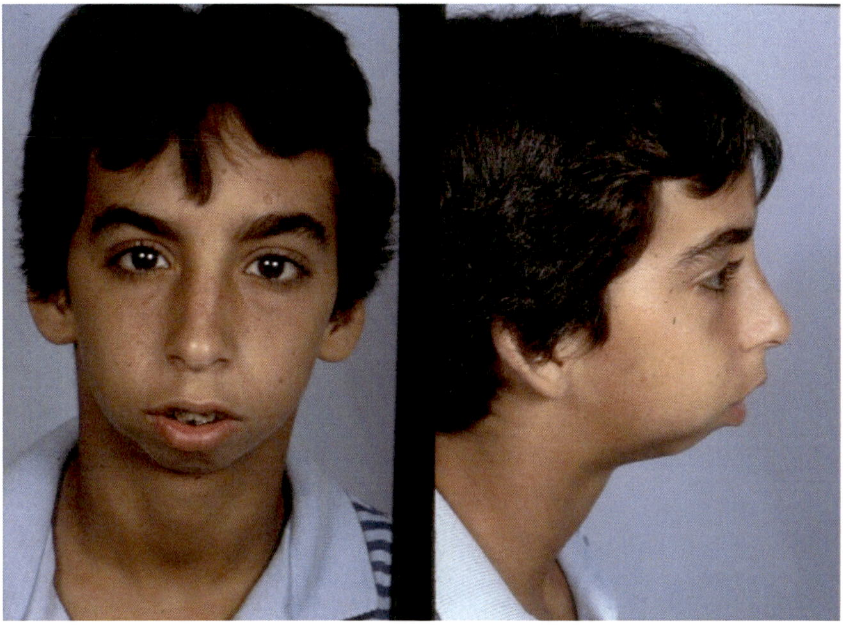

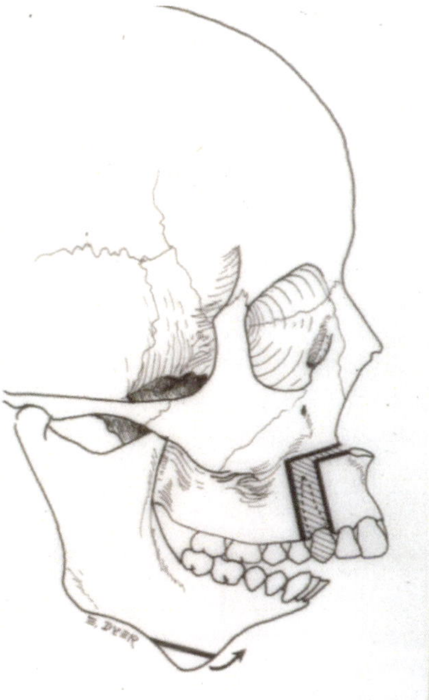

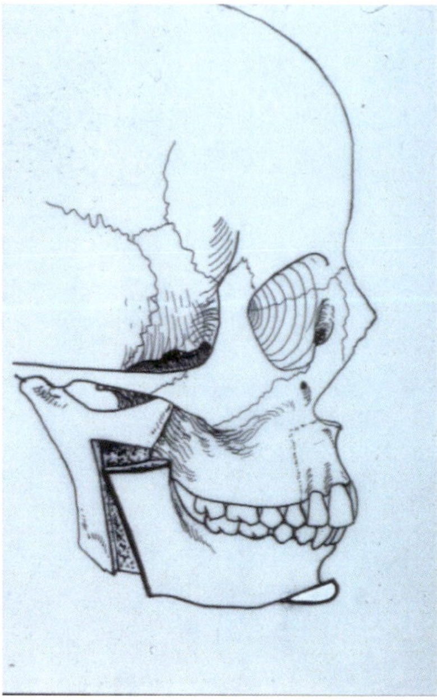

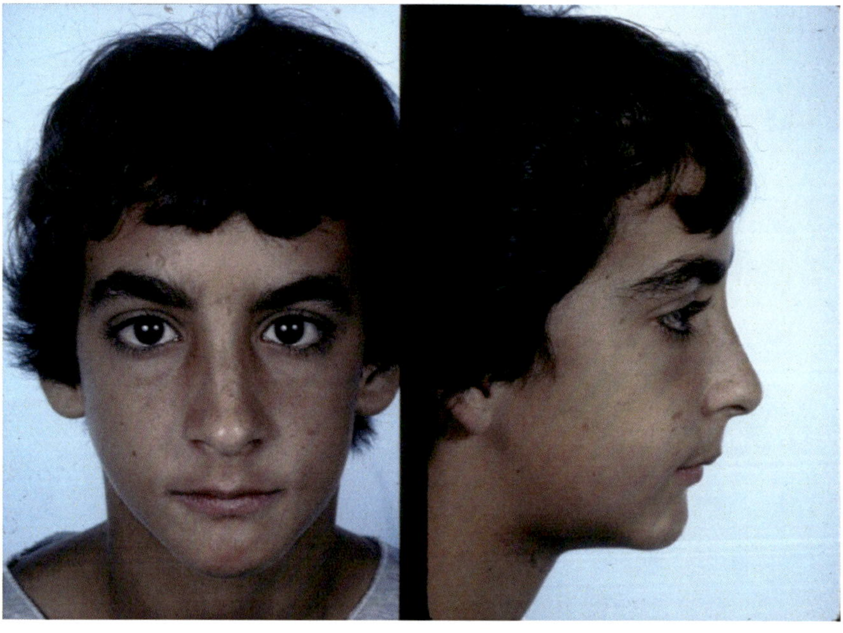

Severe case of retrogenia and long retrognathia treated with staged genioplasties, first, a jumping genioplasty along with a premaxillary set back, and second, six months later, with a mandibular advancement and a sliding genioplasty.

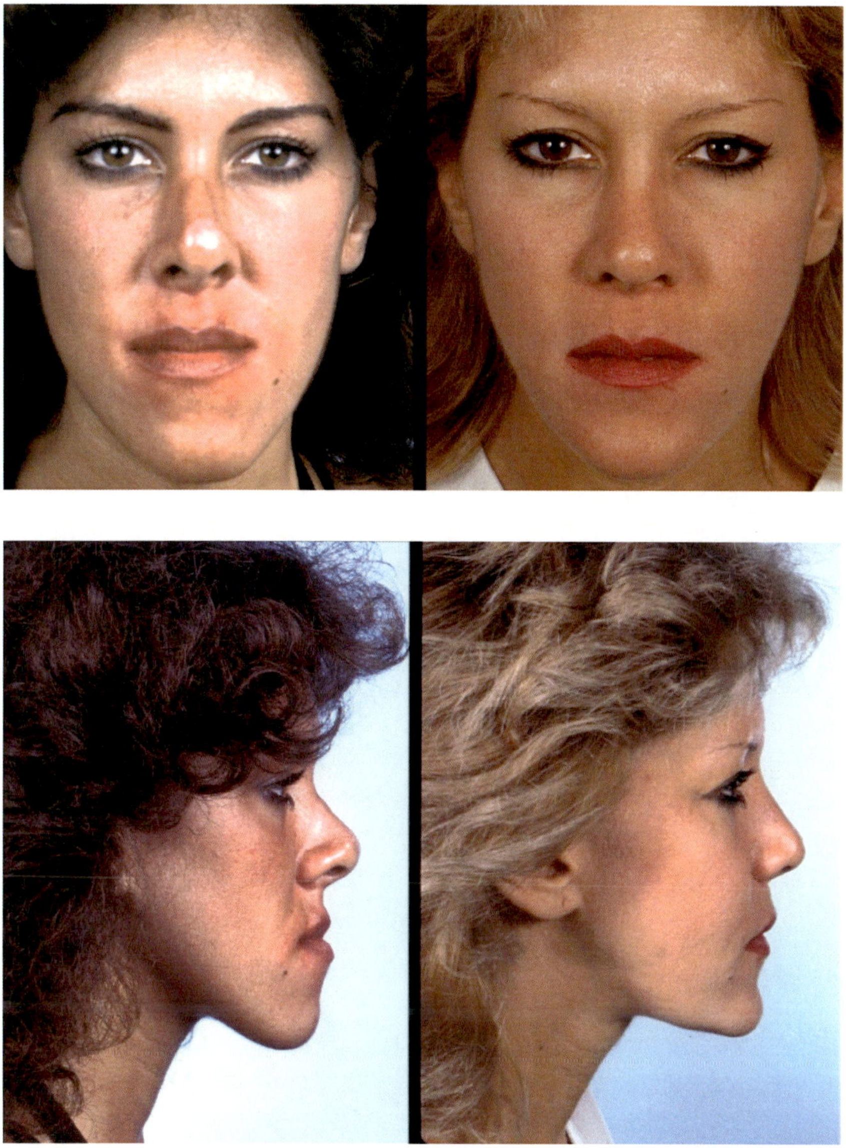

Before and after Le Fort 1 advancement, sagittal split set back of mandible and reduction genioplasty by removal of a strip of bone above the basilar segment. Also, minor rhinoplasty.

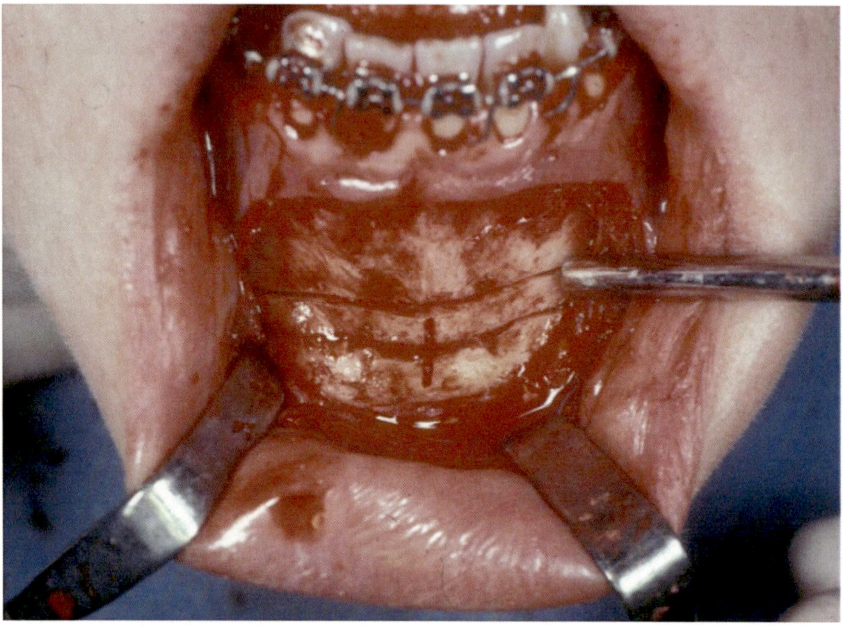

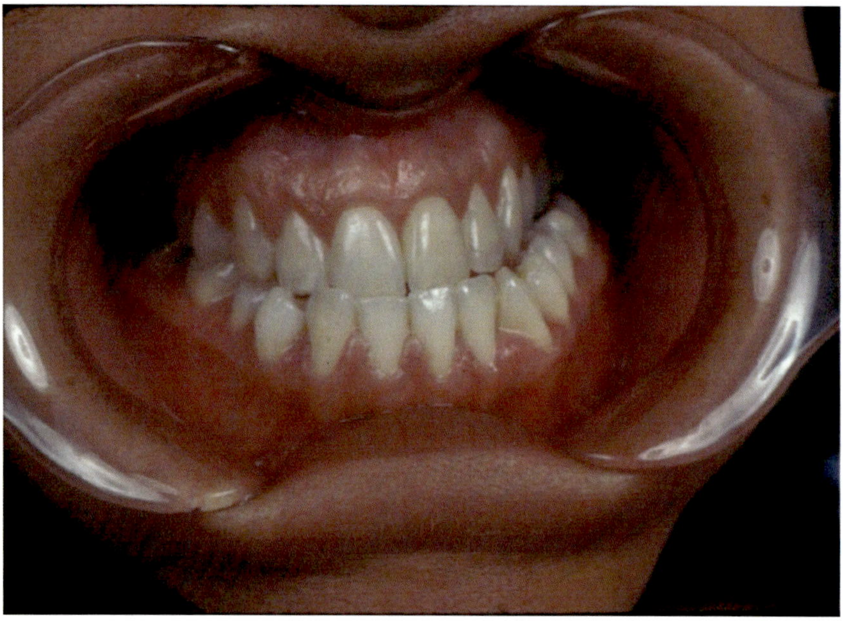

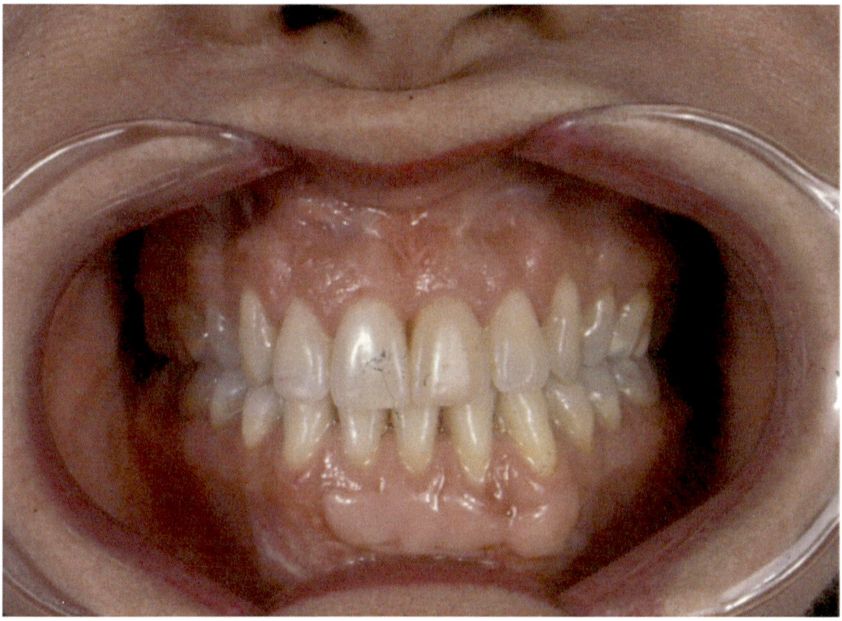

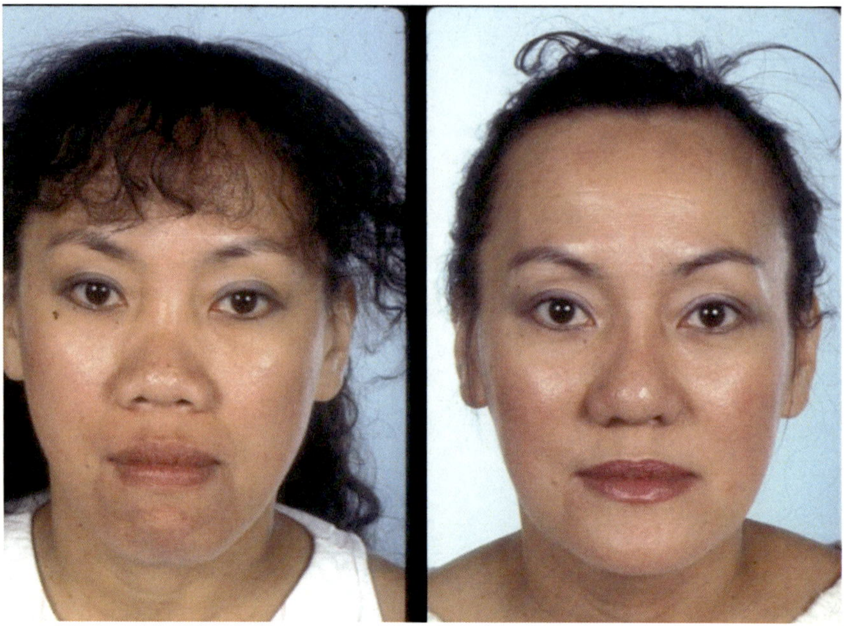

Patient of Filipino descent wished for a somewhat less Asian appearance.

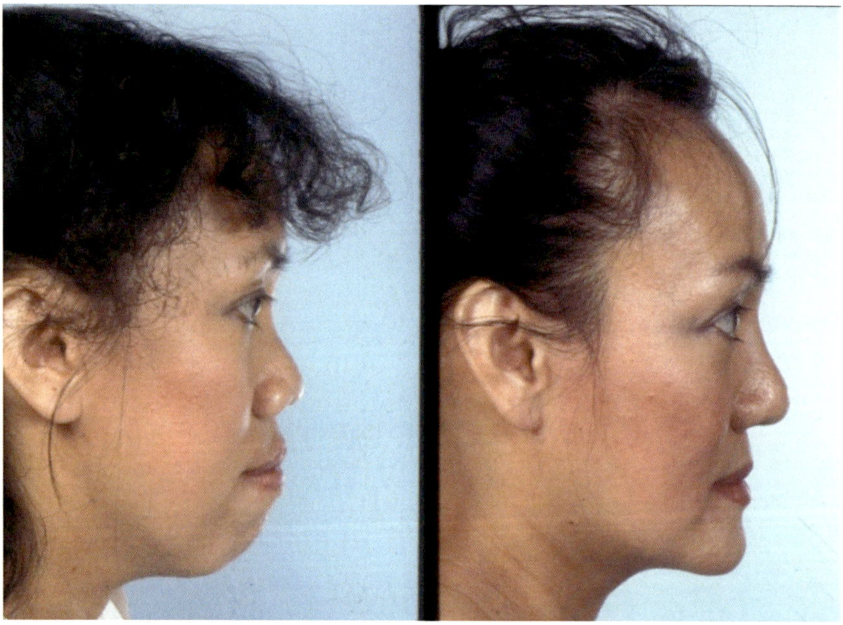

She showed bimaxillary protrusion, low nasal dorsum, and retro-macrogenia, with several missing maxillary incisors.

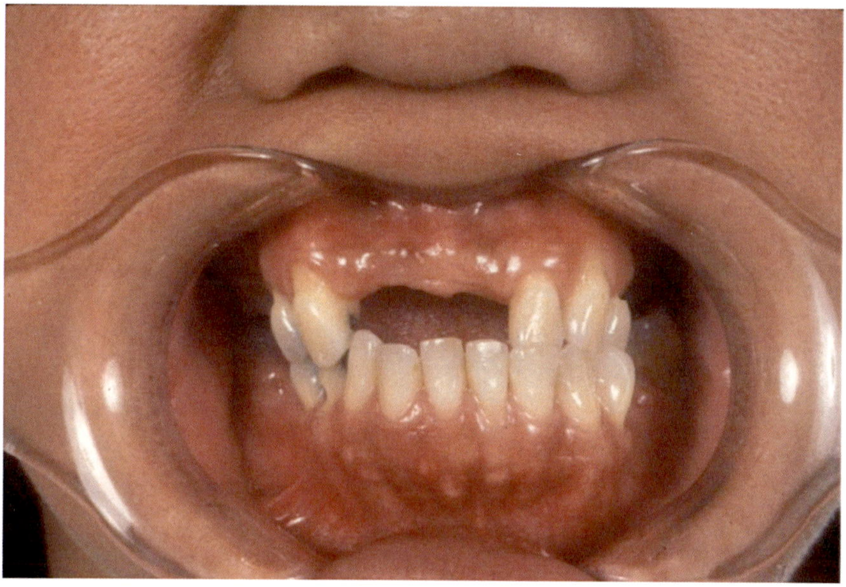

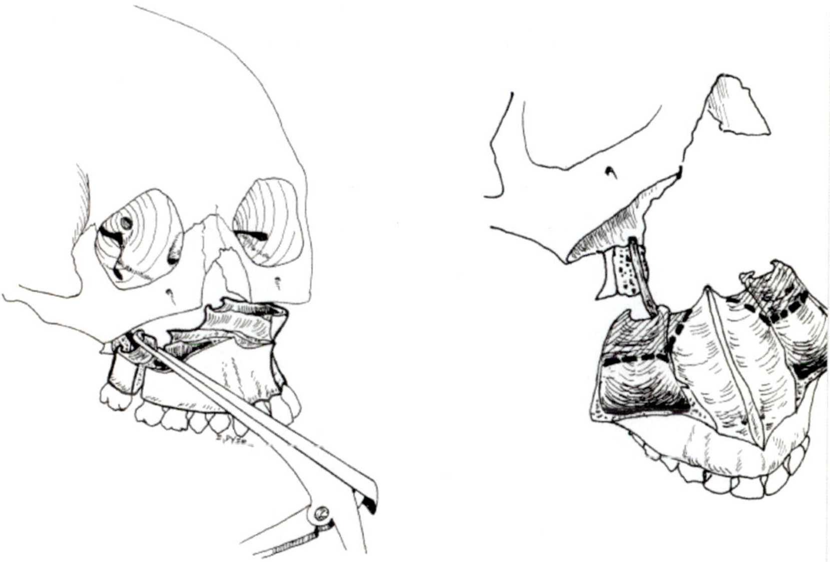

Treatment consisted of posterior displacement of maxilla after removal of third molars, while preserving the greater palatine vessels. Mandible moved back by sagittal splitting, chin reduced, and advanced, and nasal bone graft placed. She had osseo integrated implants placed where several maxillary incisors had been absent.

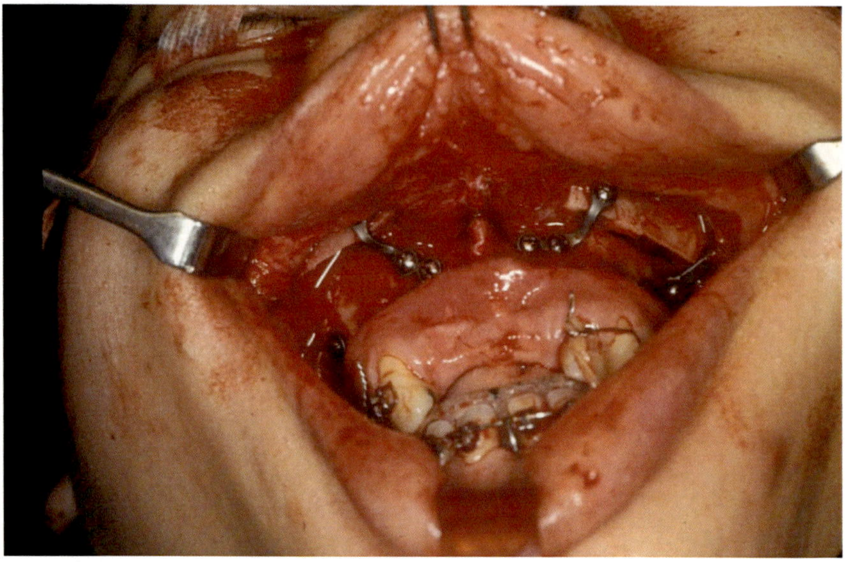

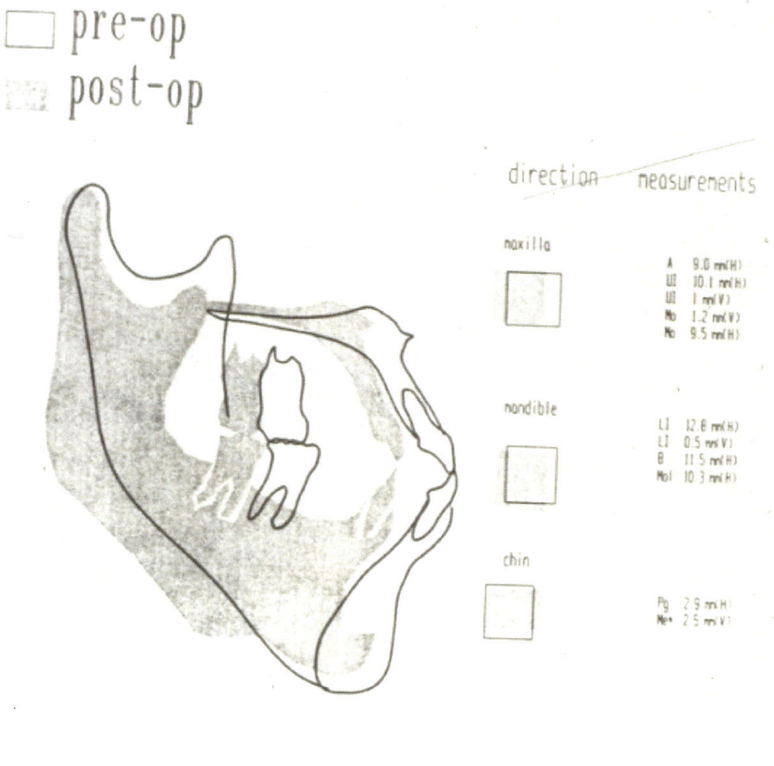
pre-op
post-op
direction
measurements
maxilla
A 9.0 mm(H)
UI 10.1 mm(H)
UI 1 mm(V)
Mo 1.2 mm(V)
Mo 9.5 mm(H)
mandible
LI 12.8 mm(H)
LI 0.5 mm(V)
B 11.5 mm(H)
Mol 10.3 mm(H)
chin
Pg 2.9 mm(H)
Me 2.5 mm(V)

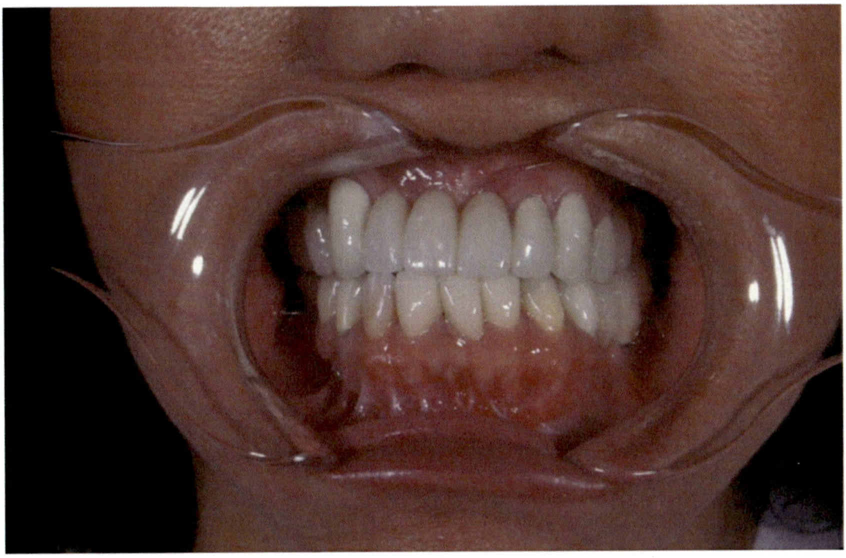

Jumping genioplasty: advance chin and
Shorten it at same time

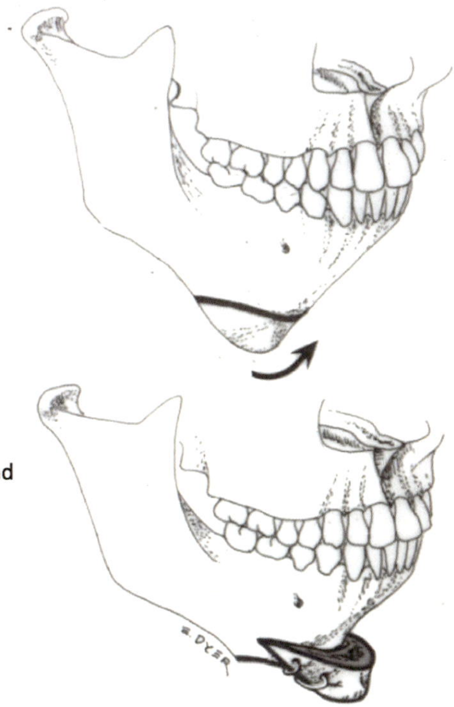

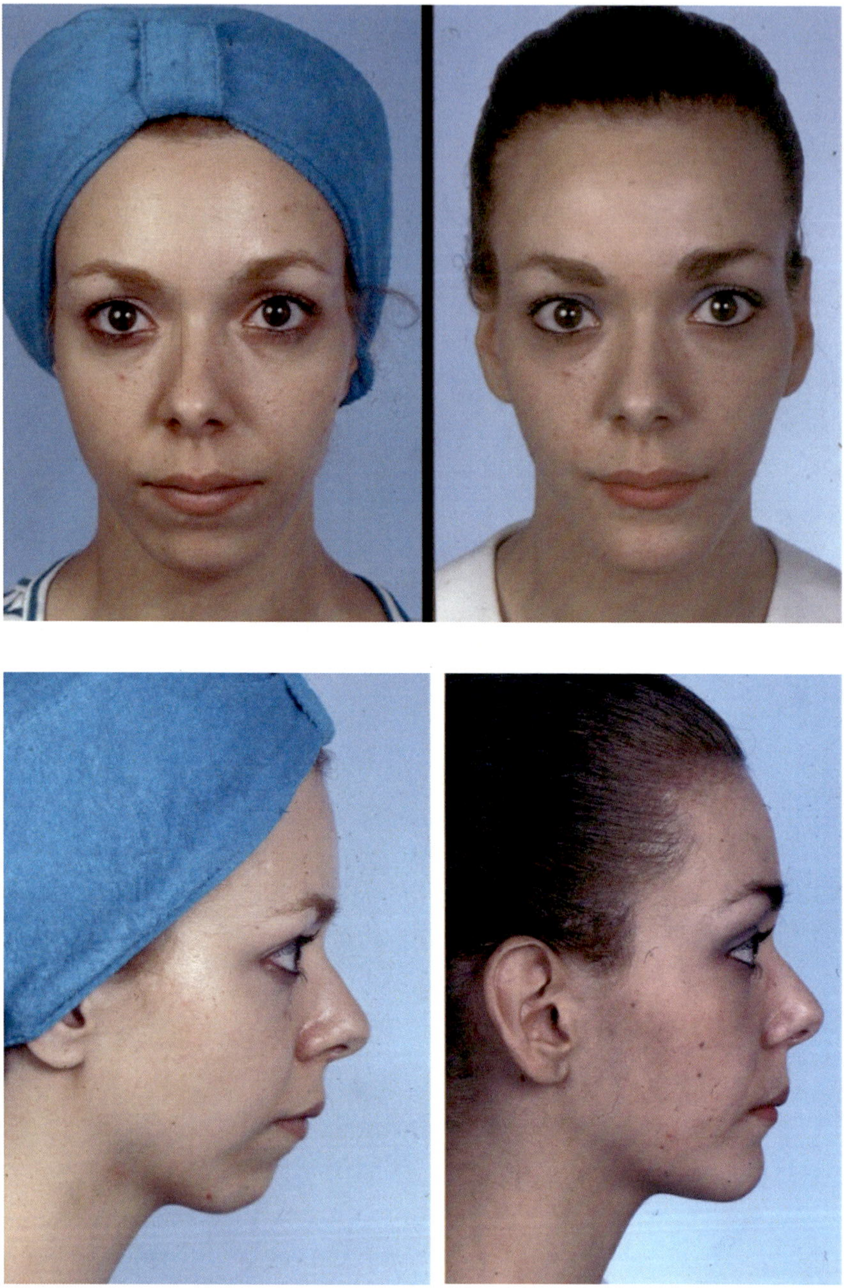

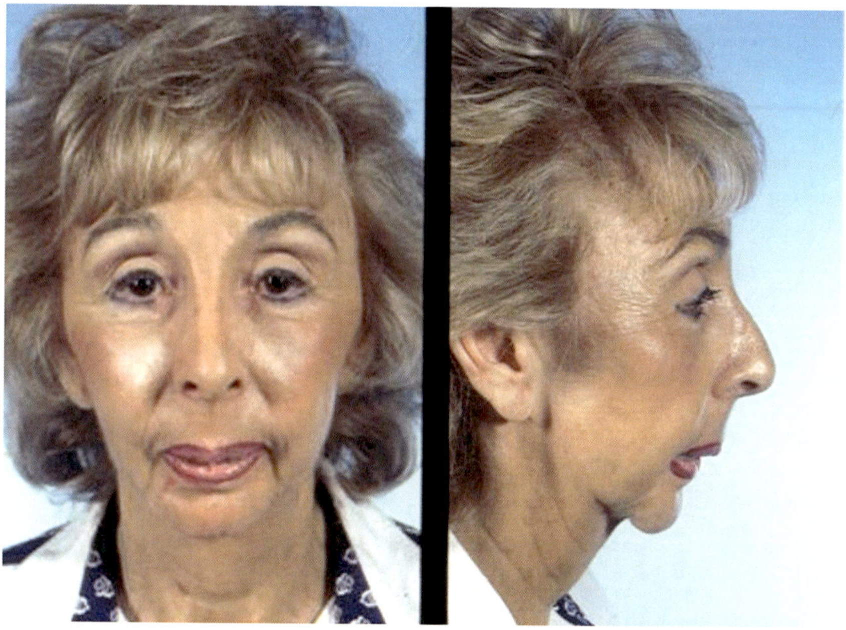

This woman was in her early 60's, and had had over 20 operations on her chin (including by Kazanjian and Ivy), with placement and extrusion of multiple types of alloplastic implants. Her chin, such as it was, was the thickness of a pencil, so there was no way to perform a genioplasty.

After a long discussion, we went ahead with an osteocutaneous iliac free flap. A skin paddle was kept to monitor the flap, and was trimmed away after several months. The bone segment from the ilium was attached to the lower border of her "pencil."

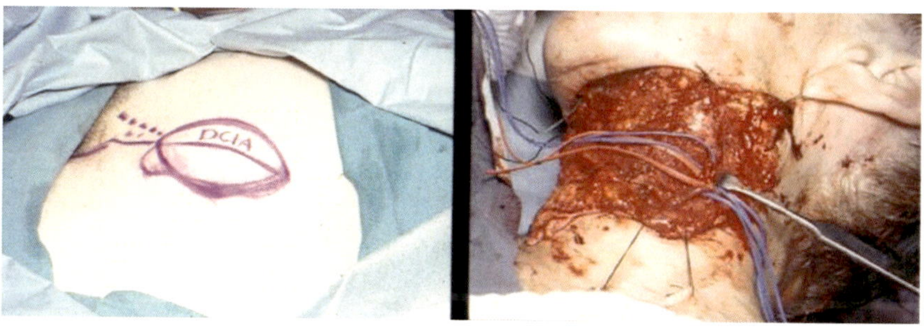

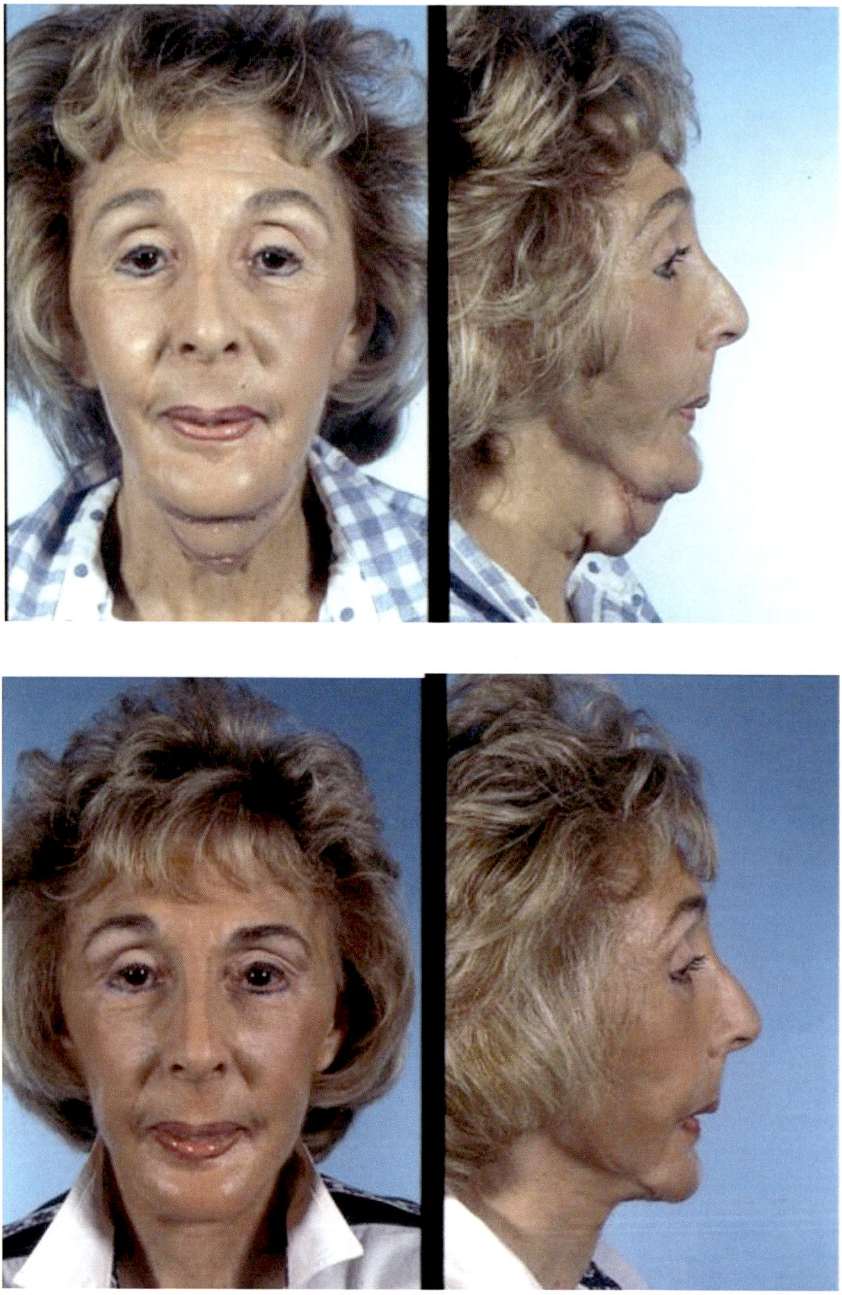

Autogenous bone

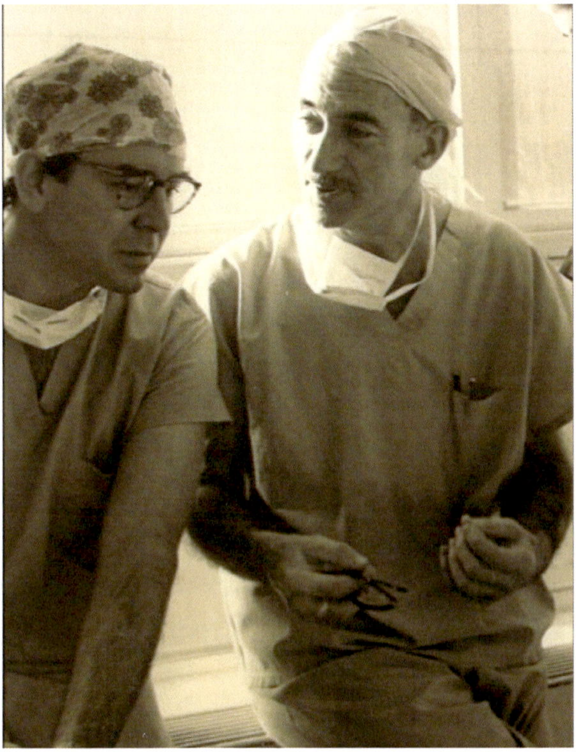

At one point early in my career Tessier is giving me advice, which may have been, "Always use autogenous bone."

There had been a paper published on cranioplasty which discussed various alloplastic materials, without any mention of autogenous bone at all.

Dr. Tessier found this annoyingly wrong, so he got a group of his trainees who he knew did a lot of bone grafting to produce what became the "Tools and Techniques." Supplement for PRS, looking at complications of bone grafting in 20,000 cases and explaining how to safely harvest cranial, iliac, costal, and tibial grafts (of which Tessier was almost the only one using them, perhaps due to his experience with Virenque). "Tools and Techniques" won the James Barret Brown award for the best paper in PRS that year.

Autogenous Bone Grafts and Bone Substitutes—Tools and Techniques: I. A 20,000-Case Experience in Maxillofacial and Craniofacial Surgery

P. Tessier, M.D., H. Kawamoto, M.D., D. Matthews, M.D., J. Posnick, M.D., Y. Raulo, M.D., J. F. Tulasne, M.D., and S. A. Wolfe, M.D.

Miami, Fla.

Summary: Alloplastic *bone substitutes* can be used to alter facial contour. In contrast, *autogenous bone grafts* have a successful 80-year history of restoring facial contour as well as the basic functional support of the craniofacial skeleton.

The traditional procedures for harvesting and using autogenous bone grafts are not obsolete. During the past 30 years, the techniques have been refined and new sources have been found, such as calvarial grafts. New tools were required and have been designed to make harvesting of grafts easier and faster for the surgeon and safer and less expensive for the patient.

Four short articles under the heading of "Techniques and Tools" are presented addressing the harvesting of (1) iliac, (2) costal, (3) tibial, and (4) calvarial grafts. These articles are based on the experience of six surgeons using the same technique and instruments in more than 20,000 autogenous bone grafting procedures. (These figures represent the group experience as of 2001. Since then, one of the junior coauthors has retired, but the remaining five continue to harvest autogenous bone grafts on a regular basis. So, the group experience as of 2004 is in the range of 23,000 procedures.) The senior surgeon's experience of 9500 procedures spans a period of 50 years (from 1946 to 1996). For the other surgeons (10,500 procedures combined), the collection period was 25 years (from 1975 to 2000). (*Plast. Reconstr. Surg.* 116 (Suppl.): 6S, 2005.)

Tools and Techniques for the Replacement of Facial Bones

Some branches of the sciences would not exist were it not for a few simple instruments. Where would astronomy be without Galileo's telescope? Where would navigation be without the compass, sextant, and Harrison's chronograph? Newspapers would not have flourished without cheap paper printed on by Gutenberg-based blocks containing Roman characters derived from the Assyrians and Phoenicians. The alphabet was easier to use and more practical than Egyptian hieroglyphs and Chinese ideograms.

Similar links can be found in medicine, such as Laennec's stethoscope for auscultation of the heart and lungs and Paré's linen vesselligatures to control bleeding. In surgery, techniques and tools are so interdependent that forging new instruments or borrowing them from other artisans always precedes the popular and widespread use of a new procedure. The development of Ophthalmology would be unimaginable without the ophthalmoscope

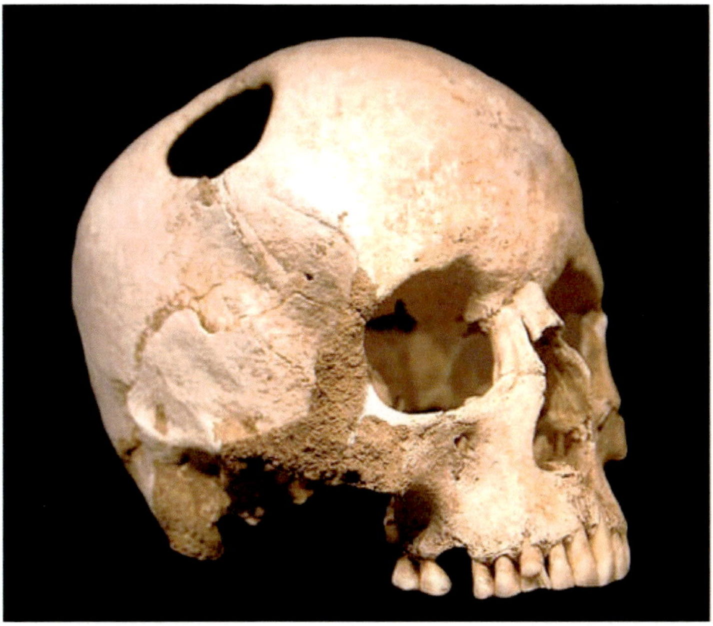

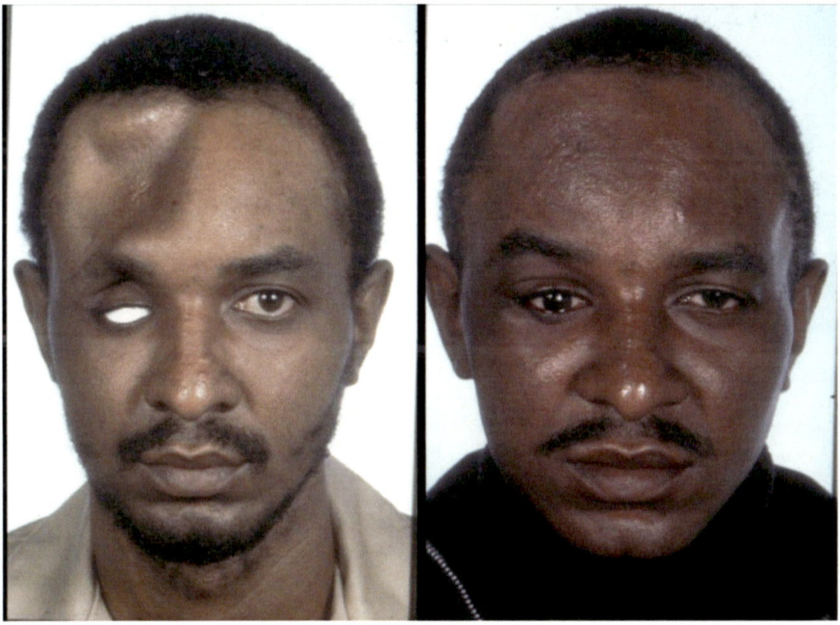

Patient with gunshot wound of the head treated by neurosurgery with significant debridement of skull. One procedure using split calvarial bone performed plus ocular prosthesis.

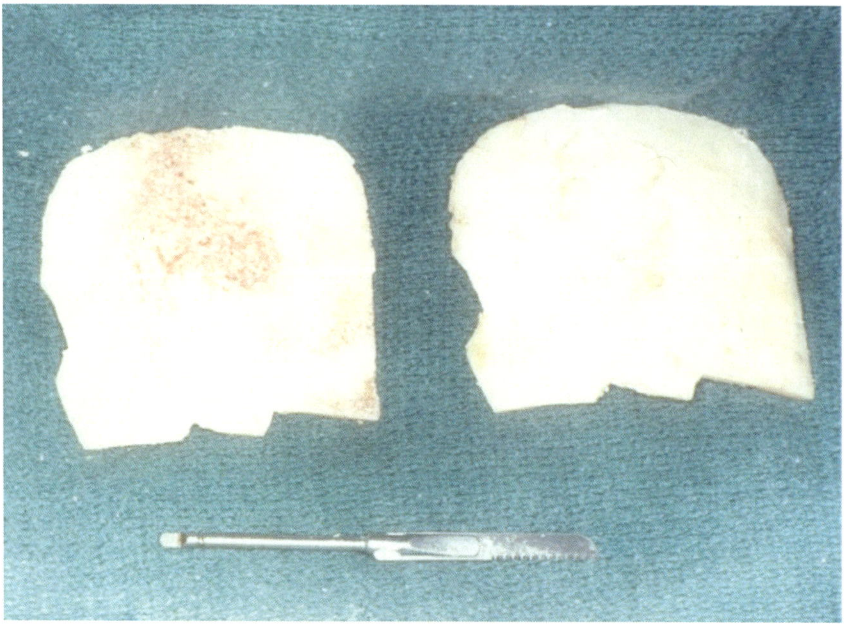

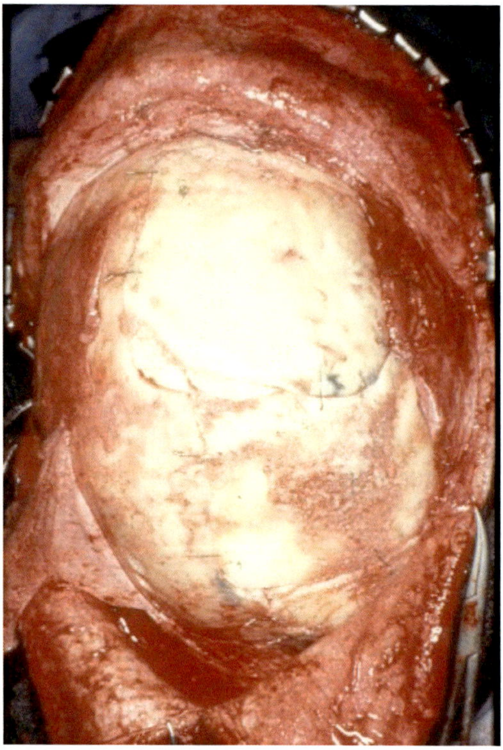

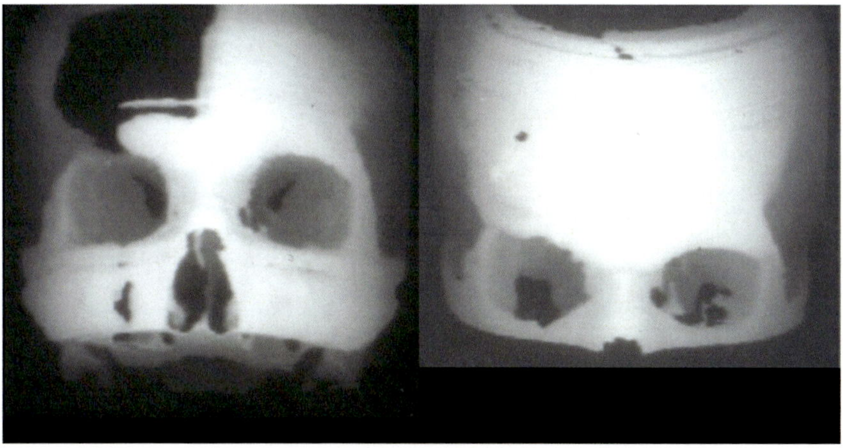

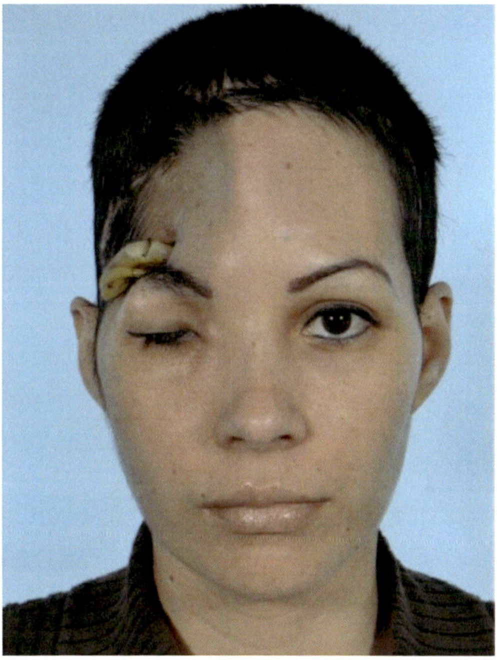

Patient shot by boyfriend in the top of head with the round going through frontal lobe and eye and orbital floor. She had had multiple procedures for persistent infection in another hospital, and arrived in our office with a drain in place which had been there for 3 weeks. We circumcised the fistulous tract, repaired the dura and covered the whole area with a latissimus free flap, a portion of which was covered with a skin graft which after a month for the flap to shrink down, was removed. The displaced zygoma was then repositioned, with an iliac bone graft to reconstruct the orbital roof and septate the orbital cavity from the cranial cavity.

Then the remnant of the muscle flap was rolled up to fill the dead space behind the superior orbital rim, and the two cranial defects corrected with split calvarial bone.

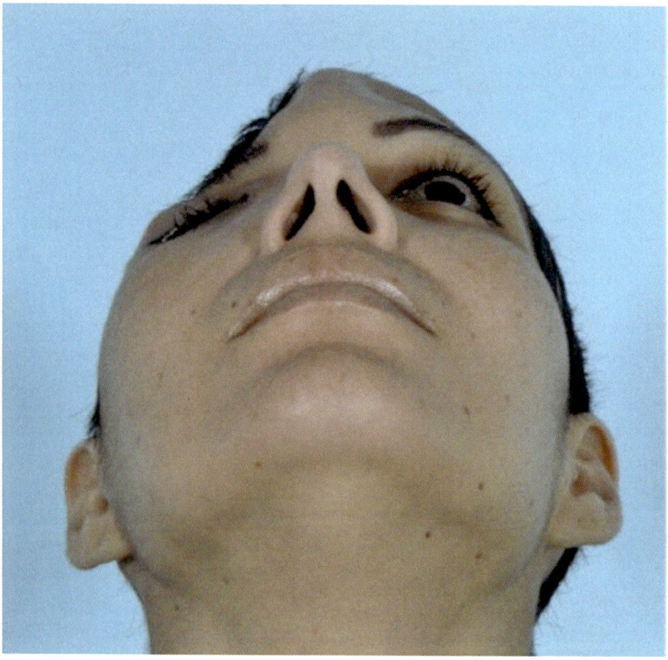

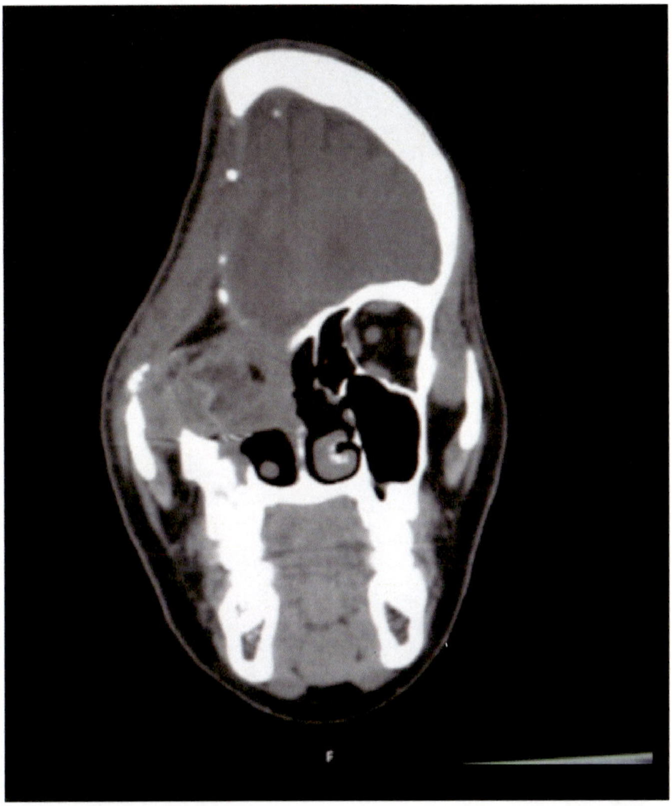

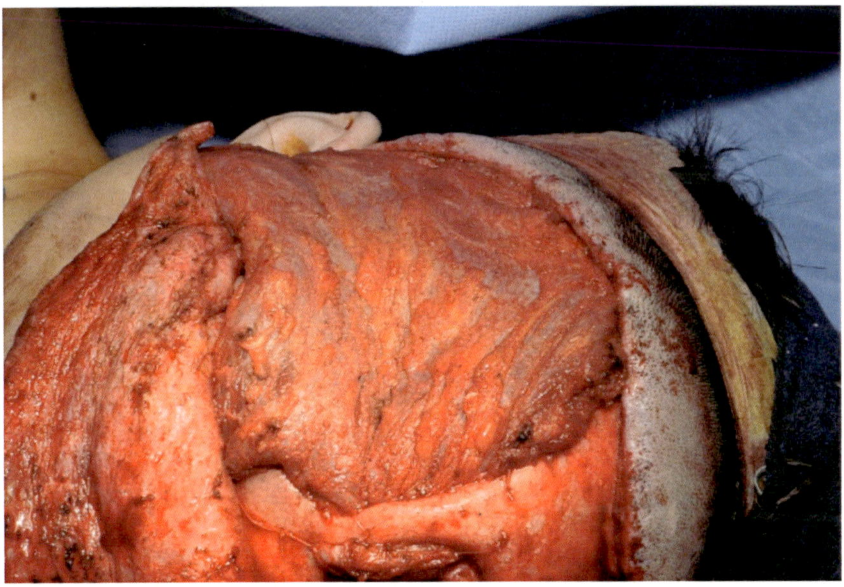

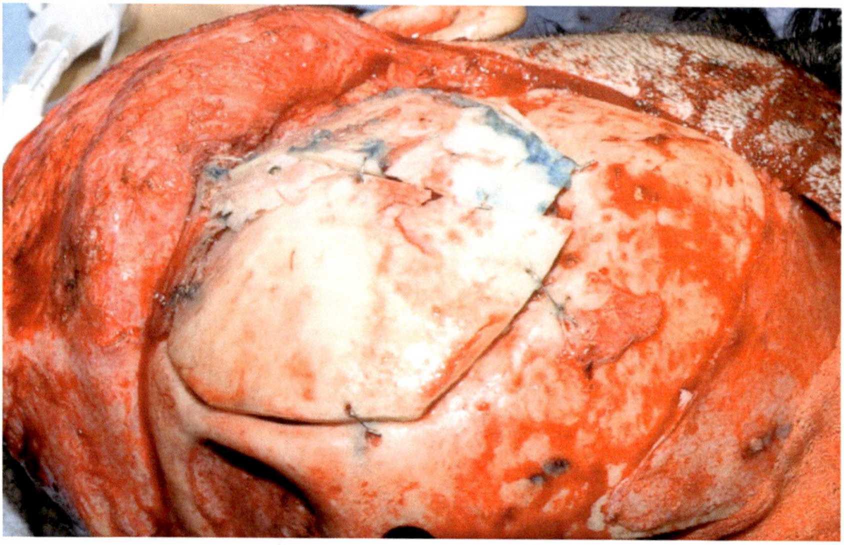

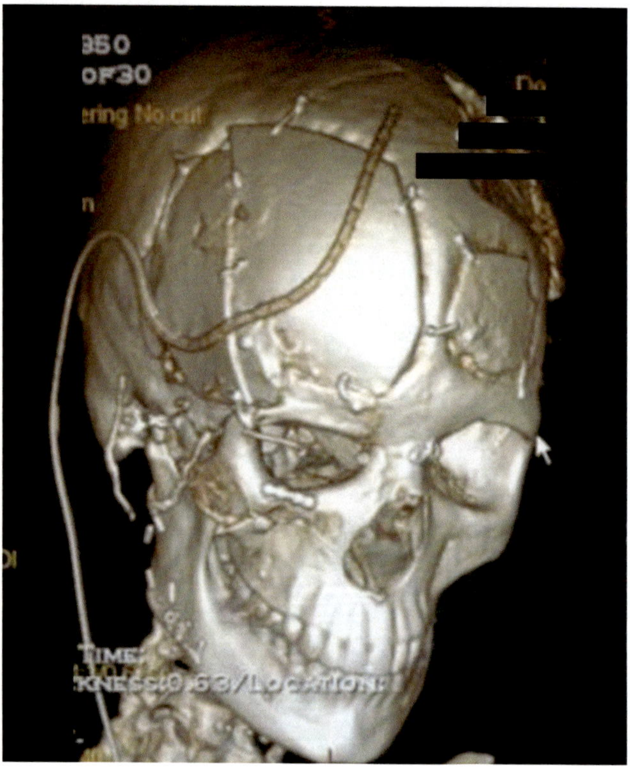

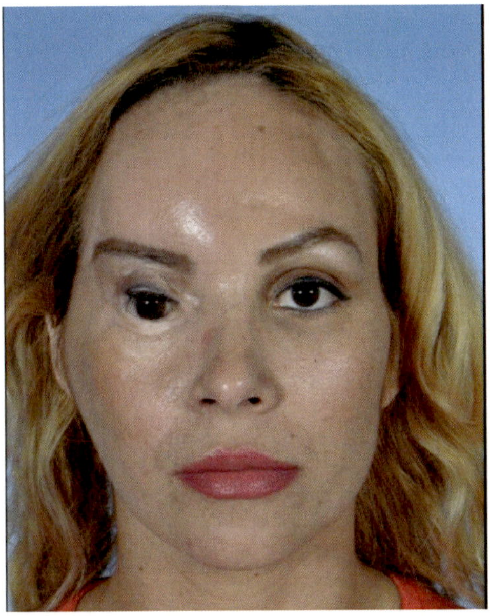

She is shown 5 years post op with no resorption of the bone, and a mediocre eye prosthesis.

PEDIATRIC/CRANIOFACIAL

Autogenous Bone Cranioplasty: Review of a 42-Year Experience by a Single Surgeon

Nicole C. Cabbad, M.D., M.B.A.
Mark W. Stalder, M.D.
Aaron Arroyave, B.S.
Erin M. Wolfe, B.S.
S. Anthony Wolfe, M.D.

Miami, Fla.; and New Orleans, La.

Background: Autogenous bone is frequently espoused as the gold standard material for cranioplasty procedures, yet alloplastic cranioplasty continues to persist in the search, presumably, for a simpler technique. Although short-term outcomes can be successful using foreign materials, long-term follow-up in these patients often demonstrates increased rates of failure because of exposure or late infection. Autogenous bone grafts, however, integrate and revascularize, and are thus more resistant to infection than alloplastic materials.

Methods: This is a retrospective review of all patients that underwent reconstructive cranioplasty for full-thickness defects, as performed by the senior author (S.A.W.) between 1975 and 2018. All procedures were performed with autogenous bone.

Results: One hundred fifty-four patients met criteria for inclusion in the report. Cranioplasties were performed for both congenital and secondary indications. Split calvaria was used in 115 patients (74.7 percent), rib graft was used in 12 patients (7.8 percent), iliac crest graft was used in 10 patients (6.5 percent), and combinations of donor-site grafts were used in 17 patients (11.0 percent). In the entire series, none of the patients suffered from complications related to infection of either the donor site or transferred bone graft. None of the patients required secondary operations to fill in defects created by the postoperative resorption.

Conclusions: Although autologous bone is widely considered the gold standard material for cranioplasty procedures, some argue against its use, mainly citing unpredictable resorption as the purported disadvantage. However, it is less susceptible to infection, and results in fewer long-term complications than alloplastic materials. There is no alloplastic material that has matched these outcomes, and thus autogenous bone should be considered as the primary option for cranioplasty procedures. (*Plast. Reconstr. Surg.* 143: 1713, 2019.)

CLINICAL QUESTION/LEVEL OF EVIDENCE: Therapeutic, IV.

This paper is unique in the literature, being a long term study of over 150 patients with cranial defects reconstructed exclusively with autogenous bone. There were NO infections and NO resorption. Since there is no similar paper available for alloplastic materials, this proves the superiority of autogenous bone. In spite of this, most defects are still treated with alloplastic materials, and one must conclude due to a lack of comfort on the part of the surgical team in harvesting and using autogenous bone.

Travels with Tessier

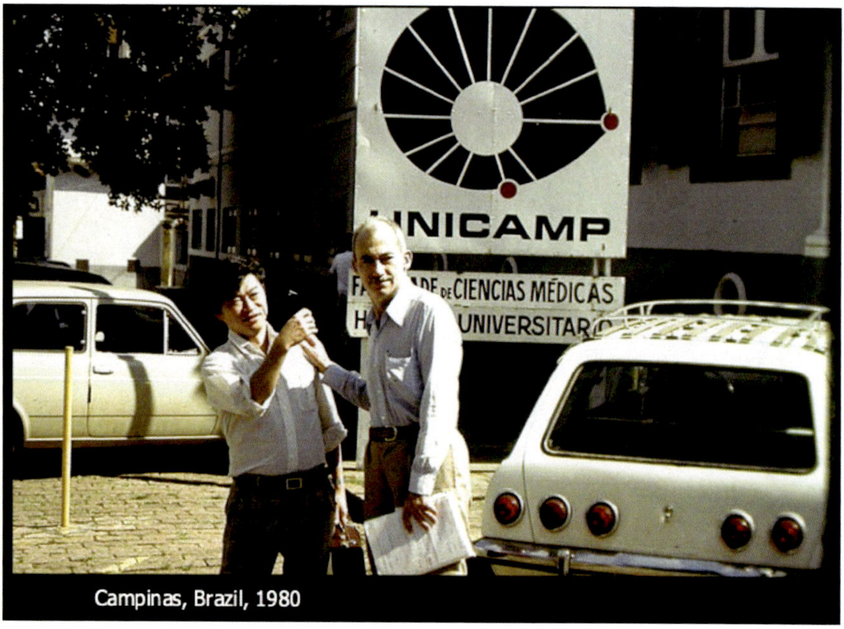

Campinas, Brazil, 1980

Cassio Raposo do Amoral spent time with Converse and Tessier and returned to Campinas to establish a Craniofacial Center in Brazil.

Henry Kawamoto and I went three times with Tessier for a week of surgery and then a week of seeing different parts of Brazil. This was the best possible type of teaching.

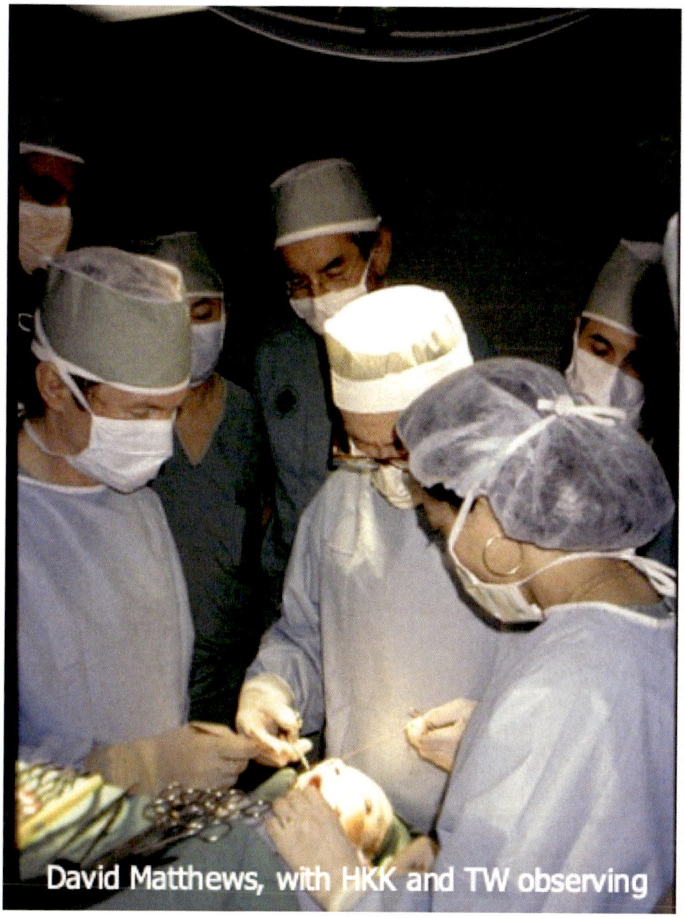

David Matthews, with HKK and TW observing

Tessier operated in a large number of American and Mexican centers. Initially Chicago, then Philadelphia, Kansas City, Louisville, Houston, Boston, San Francisco, Dallas, Mexico City, but he ended up doing the most work at Norfolk, and finally Charlotte. Cumulatively on these trips, he did more craniofacial surgery than all of the American craniofacial surgeons combined.

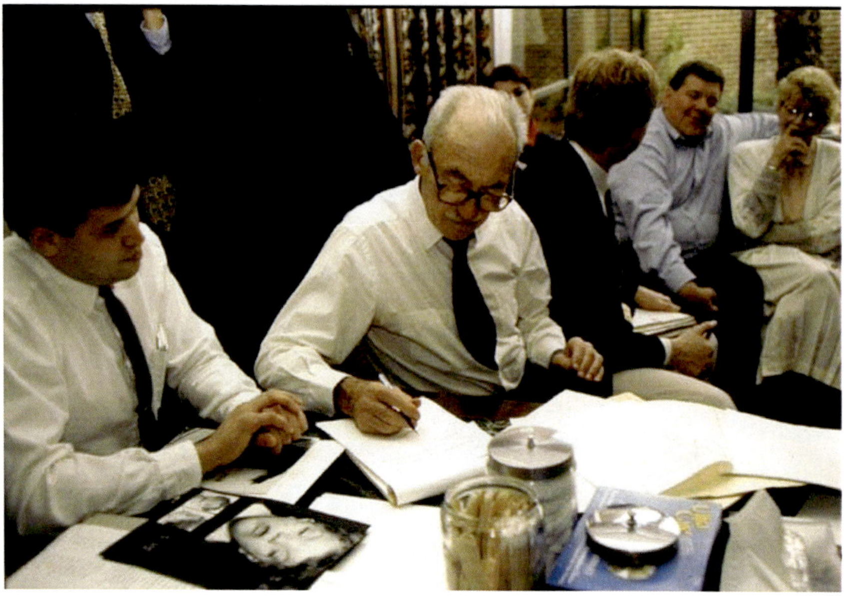

For me, the greatest learning came from watching Tessier make his notes, where he described the deformity, and his planned course of action. His notes were filled with acronyms, and one had to understand them in order to understand the notes. (For example, "CRAP" for cranial approach, "RIO" for inferior orbital rim). He also referred to other patients, i.e. voir Burgaud.

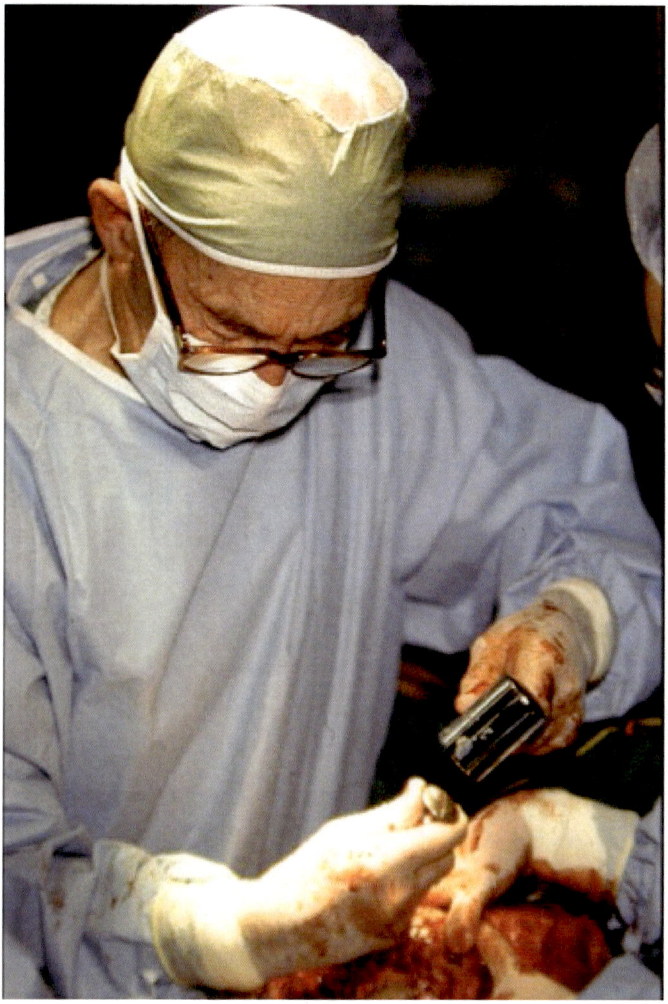

Tessier harvesting calvarial bone with a short, heavy mallet of his own design. He placed heavy emphasis on having proper instruments and sharp osteotomes and rugines (periosteal elevators).

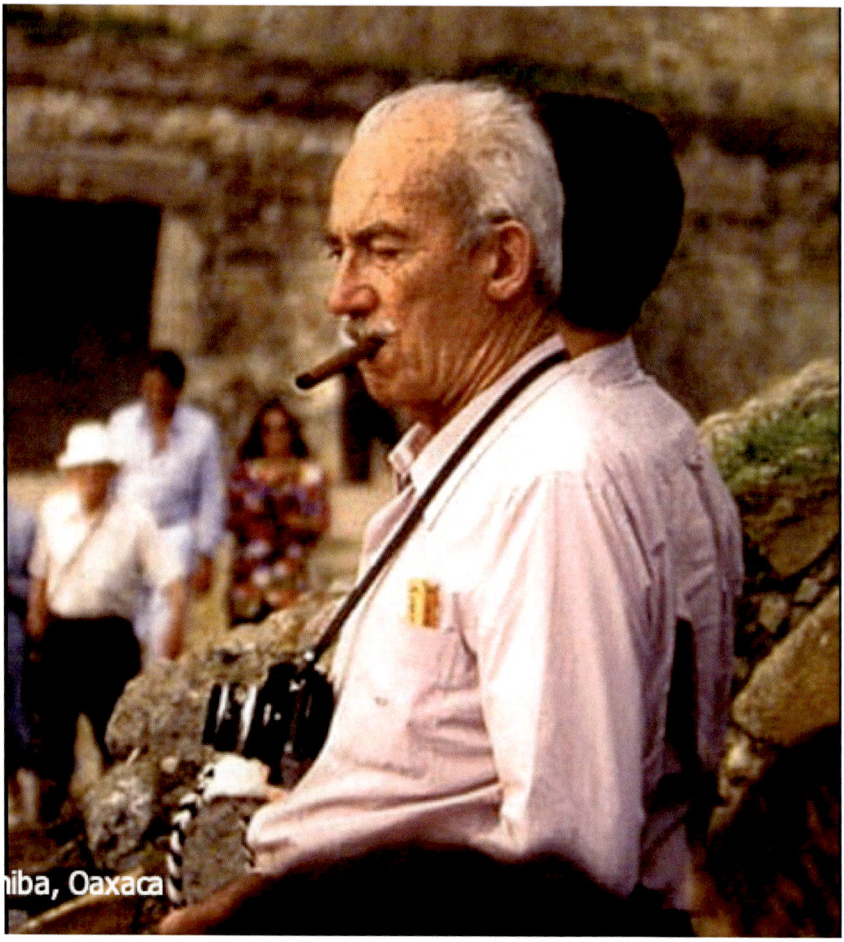

Tessier was a lover of good Cuban cigars. In the 70's, if one was in Geneva, he greatly appreciated one bringing back a box of Chateau Margaux from Davidoff. These were unavailable in France. Later the exclusive agreement with Castro was rescinded, and Cohibas became available in France.

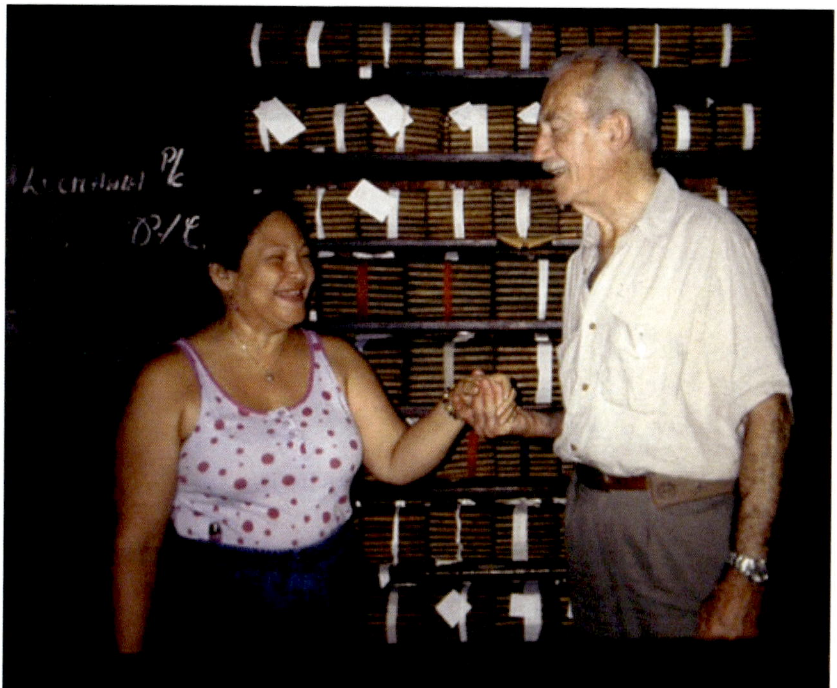

In the Partegas factory vault, Havana

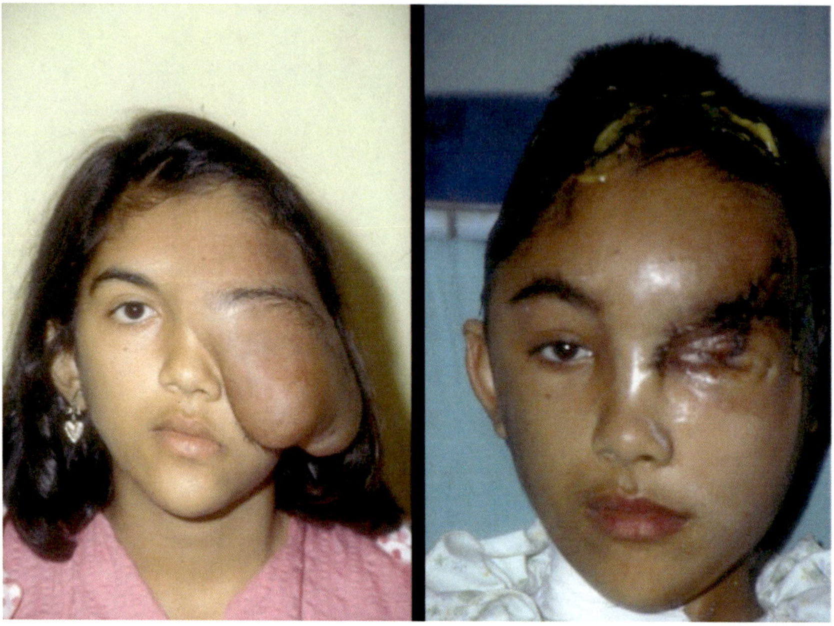

Patient with orbital neurofibromatosis operated on in Cuba by Tessier and his team. Patient shown two days post op. Henry Kawamoto was sent to the ilium to harvest two large grafts for orbital floor and roof and Tessier did all of the excision, including the intracranial portion. I assisted.

Hopefully she was able to get an ocular prosthesis for the missing eye.

S.A.P.P.

Dr. Tessier's office for most of his career was in 25 Avenue Kleber, several blocks from the Etoile. It was on the second floor of an old white stone building, and the family quarters were around the back of the patient area. Dr. Tessier had bought a plot of land in the Saint Germaine area, rural country outside of Paris, and had plans drawn up for a house. His wife, Mireille, felt that this would be too far away from Paris, so they searched for an apartment in Paris, and found one on Boulevard d'Auteuil in Boulogne, just across the street from the Roland Garros Tennis Stadium where the French Open was held. The two story apartment had been previously owned by the actor, Omar Sharif. Tessier, ever fond of acronyms, referred to it as SAPP - Stupide Apartment Parisianne de Prestige.

On the second floor there was a study and file room where Tessier stored his records, and the Tessiers were gracious in letting me go through the records to find cases with good before and after images. I stayed in the guest room downstairs and started at 7 am, often going on until dinner for most of a week, four or five times over a year period.

The result was a long PowerPoint showing Tessier's results over three periods: 1945 to 1956 (mostly burns and late facial trauma), 1956 to 1968 (early days of craniofacial surgery), and 1968 until mid 1990s (the *mise au point* of craniofacial surgery, including the monobloc frontofacial advancement. The PowerPoint, entitled "Long London" was shown in a continuous loop at the London Meeting.

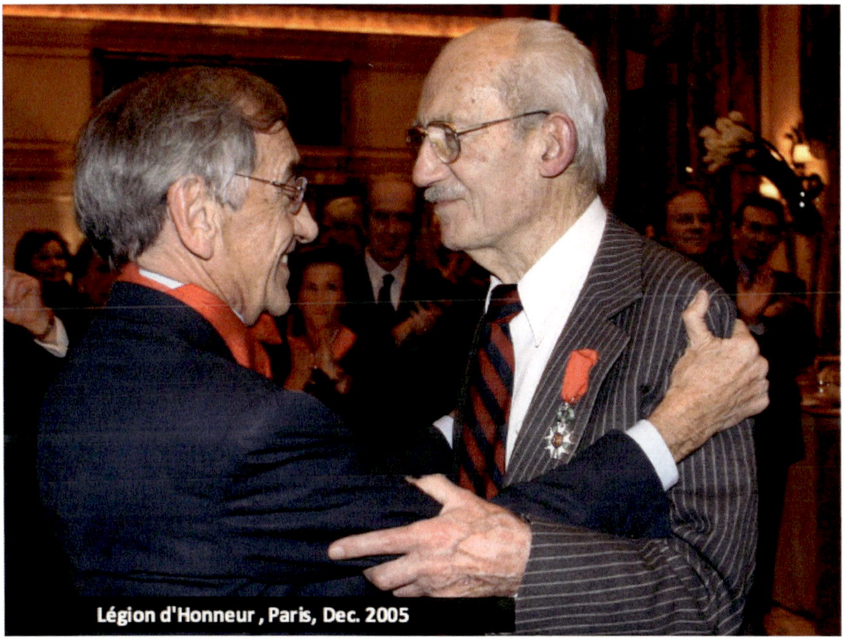
Légion d'Honneur, Paris, Dec. 2005

Finally, in 2005 Tessier received the Legion d'Honneur, long overdue. He had received every honor available except in France where he was still considered an outsider by the Parisian elite, perhaps since his background and training had been in Britain and not Paris. Parisians can be snobs.

When Jacqueline Auriole, an aviatrix and daughter of the French President, crash landed her plane in the Seine in 1949, she sustained a comminuted Le Fort 3 fracture. She was hospitalized at Hôspital Foch, and a number of "expert" plastic surgeons were asked to see her. One, who was a rhinoplasty doctor, recommended a rhinoplasty!

She was on the service of Tessier's old nemesis, Ginestet.

Nothing was being done for the patient, someone told the family that they should ask for a consultation with Tessier. This was, perhaps begrudgingly, allowed by Ginestet.

Tessier said that she needed reduction of her fractures, proper fixation, as well as bone grafting for her flail maxilla. Ginestet was able to prevent her being cared for by Tessier by sending her to New York where she was treated by John Converse. (22 operations).

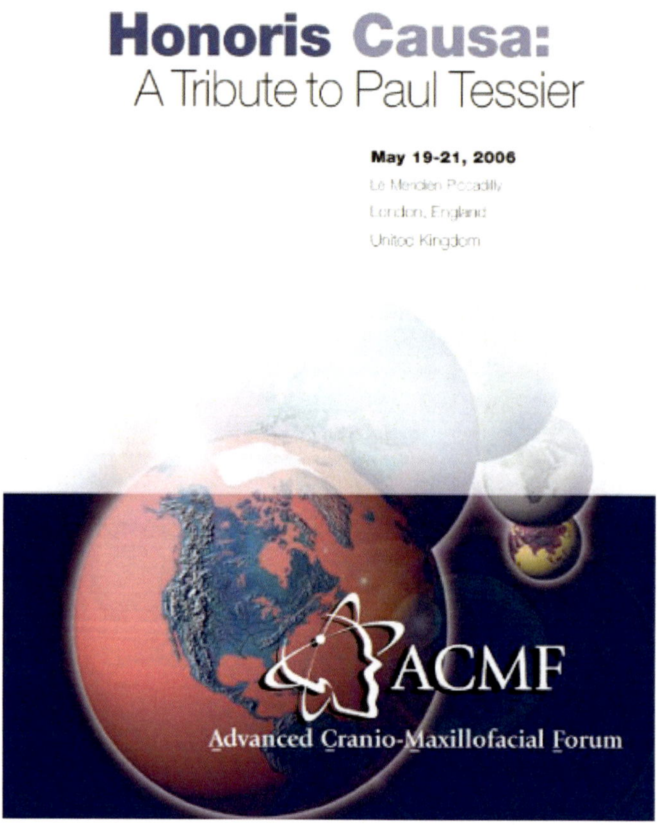

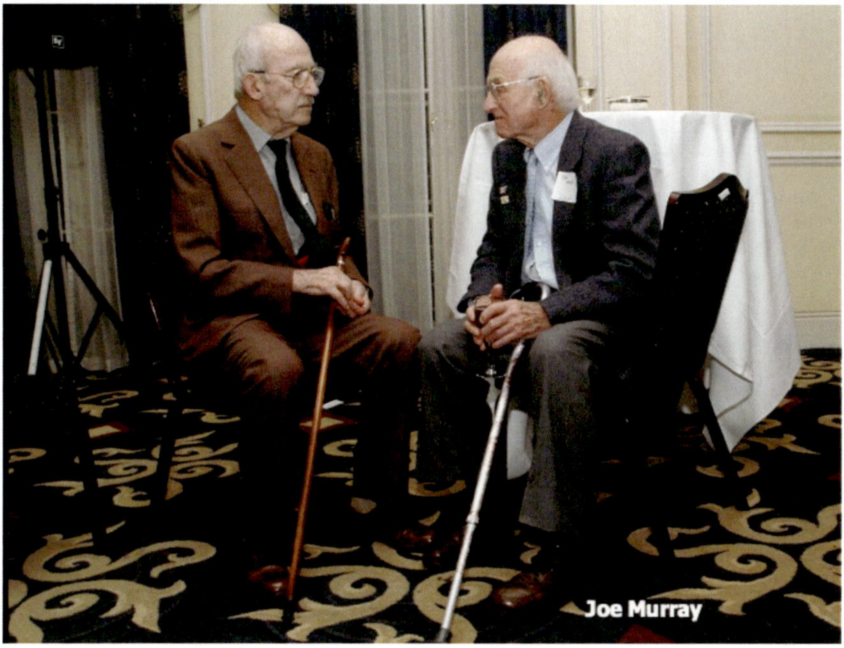

Joe Murray

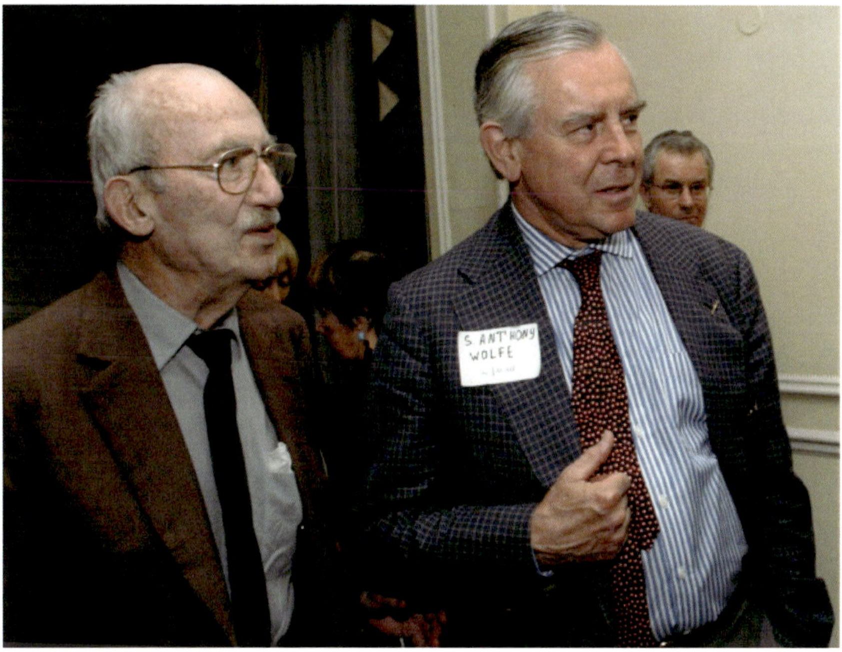

DOCTEUR PAUL TESSIER

5/28/07

26, BOULEVARD D'AUTEUIL
92100 BOULOGNE
TÉL. 01 46 04 81 80
46 04 81 10

Mon cher Tony,

Je vous remercie de l'affectueux message envoyé à Mireille et qui me concerne aussi.
Comme toujours, ça a été un plaisir de vous avoir dans la maison travaillant dans VOTRE bureau. Qu'y avez-vous grappilié de nouveau ? Vous n'y avez pas tout exploré et vous pourrez encore vous distraire cet automne après votre présidence au Congres de Bahia.
Vous avez laissé vierges dix sujets...

1- Les 14 Chapitres du livre préparé jusqu'en 1982 et prêts à partir chez l'éditeur.
2- 2-Une grosse liasse de feuilles de diapos pleine de Fentes et d'AGENESIES prêtes à vous servir pour VOTRE C.A.A.C (mais il n'y a pas les C.T correspondants)
3- 3-plusieurs liasses d'Esthétique qui ne sont pas tous indifférents.

Ailleurs j'ai retrouvé :

4- Le canthus externe,(totalement écrit en anglais)

5- Ma dermo mastopexie totalement écrite. Vous ne saviez pas que je me suis beaucoup intéressé aux seins (dont Françoise et Madeleine Lejour disaient qu'ils étaient les plus beaux du monde... ?)

6- La TMJ ankylosis (à ma façon)

7- Une ébauche sur 7 cas (E.S.F.)

8- Une nouvelle toute nouvelle approche de la D.O.G (intéressante me semble-t-il)

9- Vous pouvez aussi vous amuser sur mes 50 ou 70 crânes et leur trouver un riche acheteur(il y a deux cas dont je ne sais s'ils sont des Neandertal ou de grands primates actuels...)

Une autre fois vous pourrez vérifier comment les transferts de 50 ou 100 C.T ont été faits par nos radiologues (ERNEST et COQUILLE) d'analogique en numérique et s'ils vous semblent utilisables pour VOTRE C.A.A.C.
La prochaine fois nous ferons un livre avec tous ces matériaux

Avec vos débauches de Londres je crains que vous n'ayez épuisé les trésors de publicité de STRYKER-LEIBINGER.

Aimez-vous bien votre Ambroise PARE. Y en a-t-il un autre à MIAMI ?

Toutes nos amitiés à vous à Derdree et vos six petits

This letter from May 28, 2007, is a list of projects Tessier is charging me to finish. Unfortunately, I have failed to do most of them, publishing his paper on the Baron-Tessier flap (subcutaneous island flap of clavicular skin) and the Arrhinias.

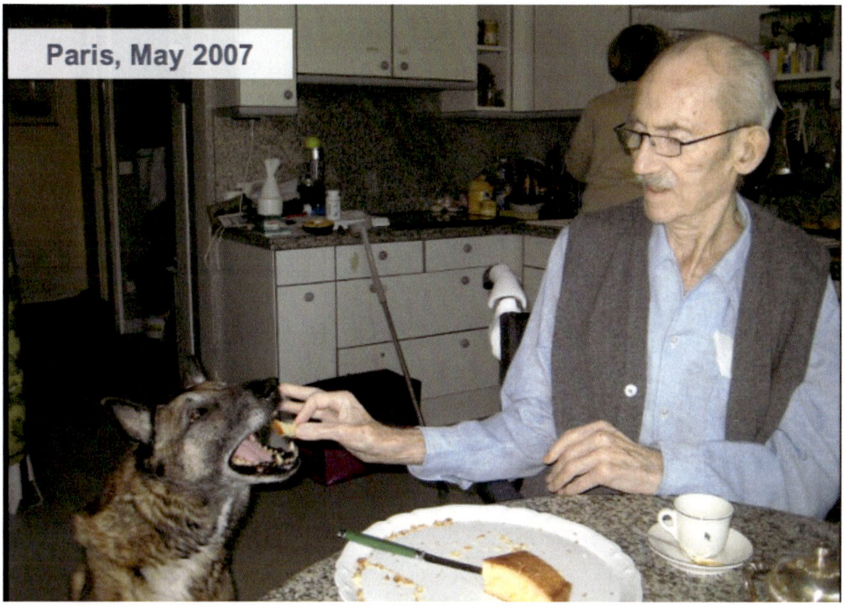

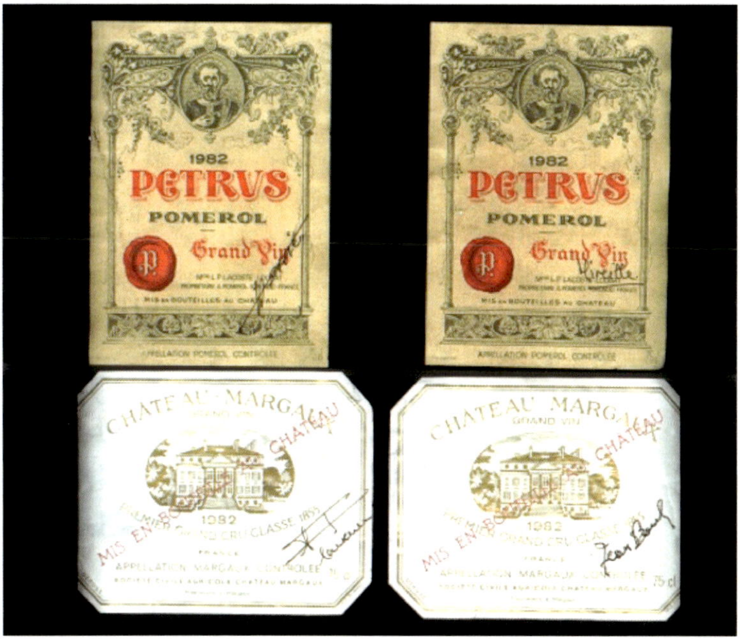

This was a present from the Tessiers. I had dinner with Paul, Mireille, Laurence, and Jean- Paul one night, and they steamed off the labels of the four bottles of wine that the four of us consumed and signed them. I hesitate to place a value on these four bottles.

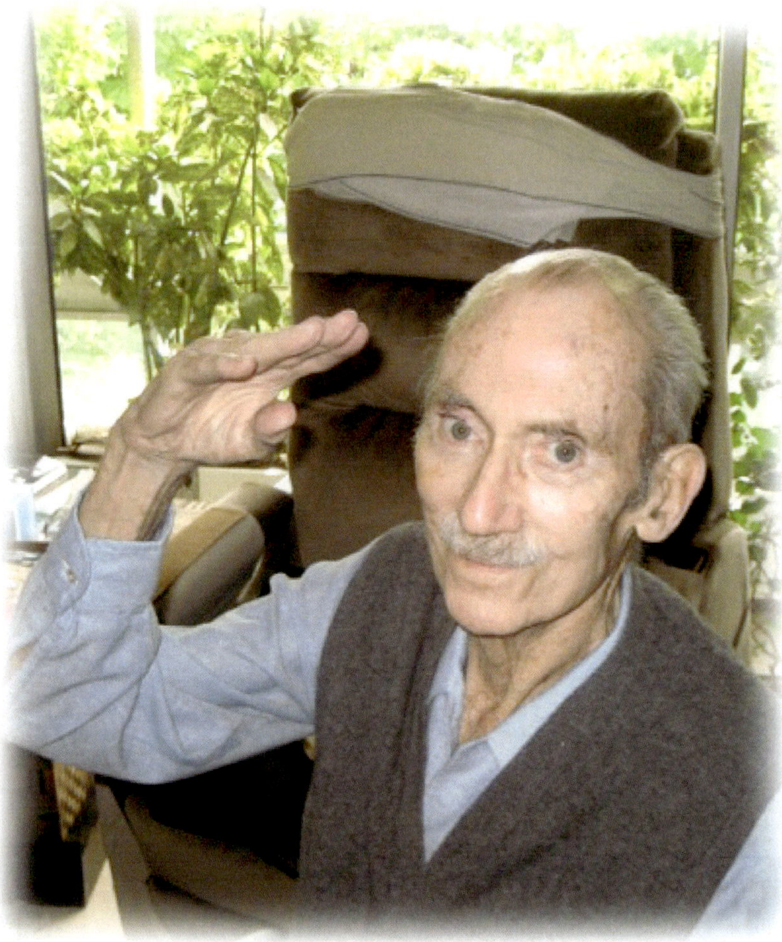

Tessier saluting his surgical children and grandchildren attending the International Society of Craniofacial Surgery meeting in Bajia, Brazil, in 2007 where I was President. This is the last photo I have of him.

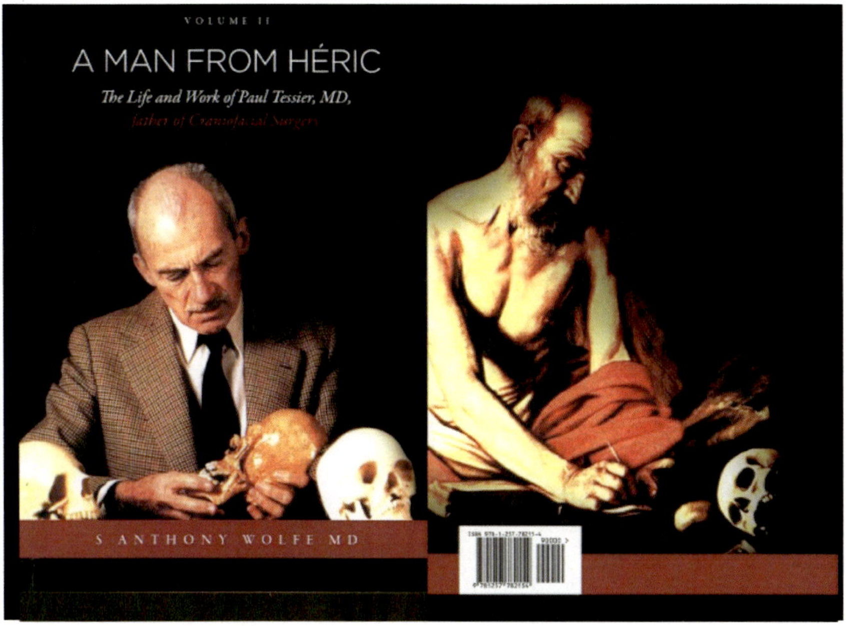

My biography of Tessier, which would never have been possible without the generosity of his wife, Mireille, and many of his friends and trainees.

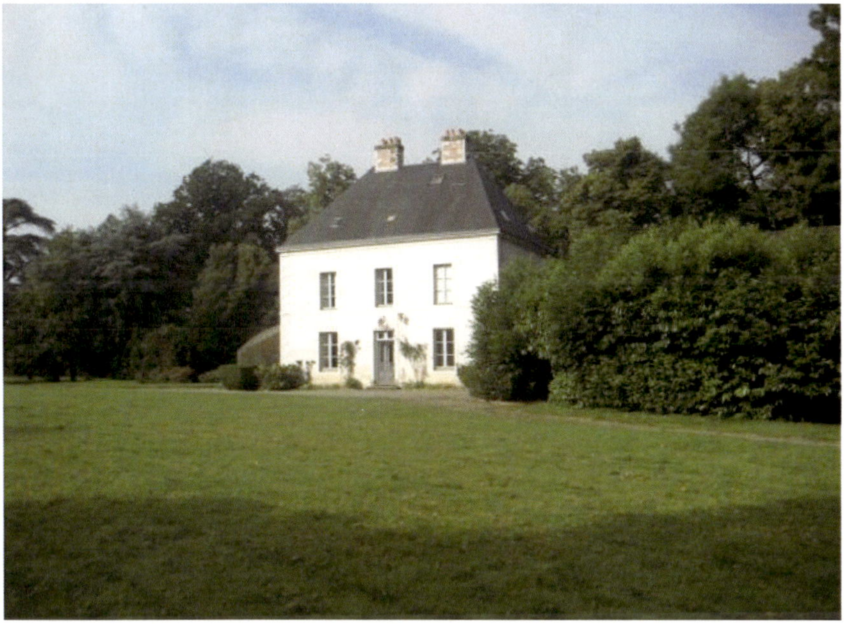

Bonne Hygié, the Tessier/Clergeau home built by his grandfather Auguste Clergeau.

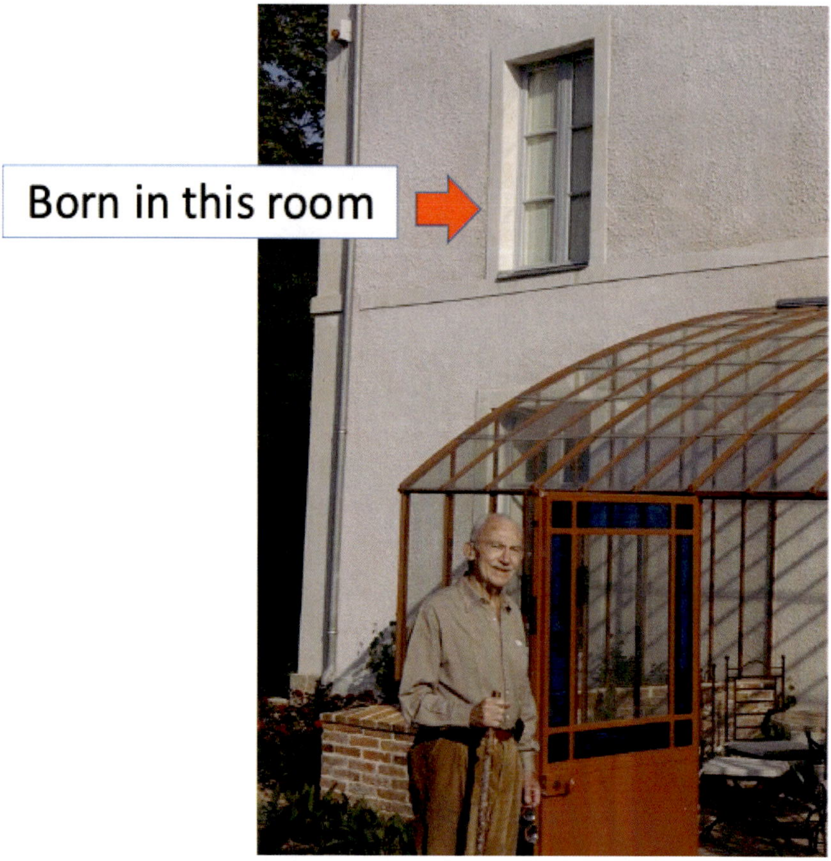

Paul and Mireille and their Alsatian.

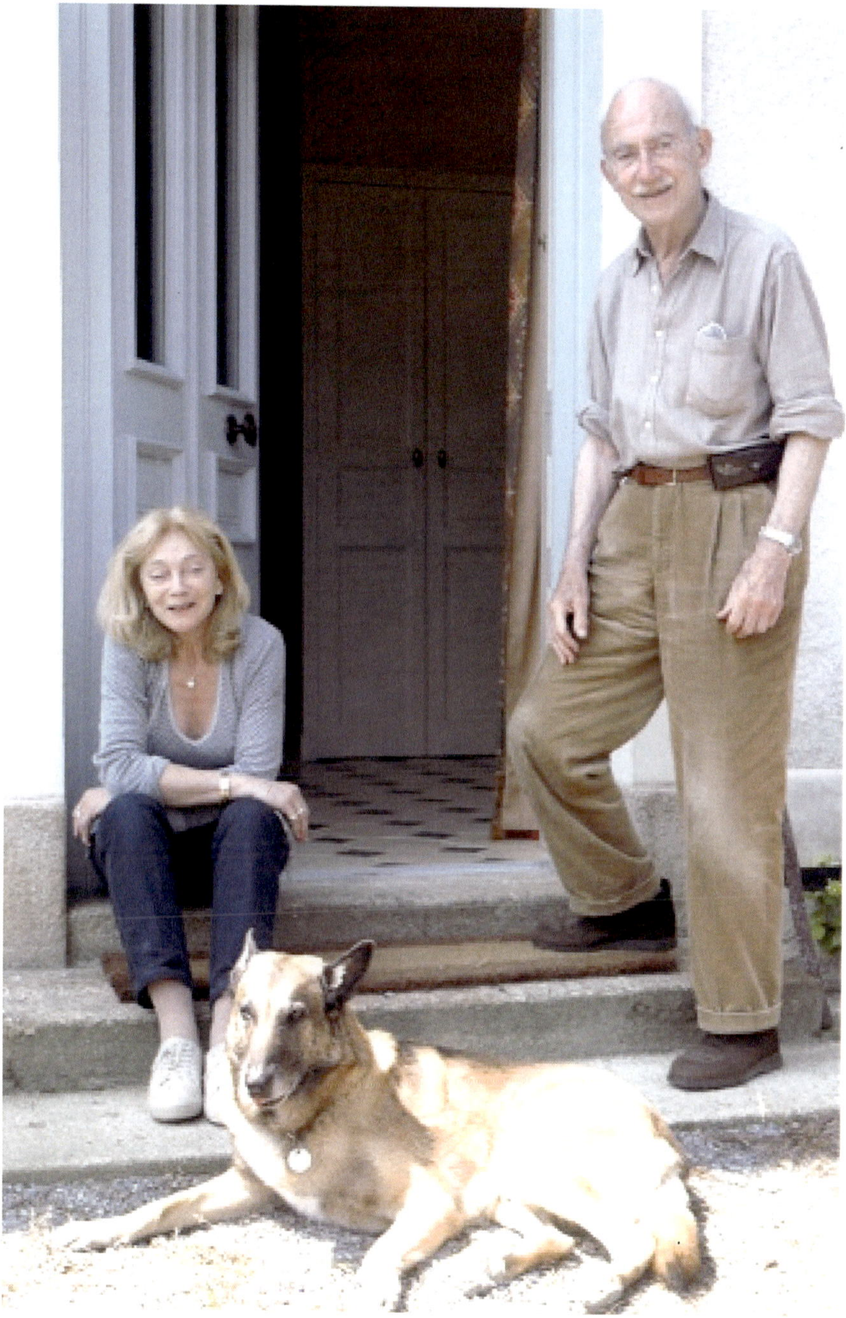

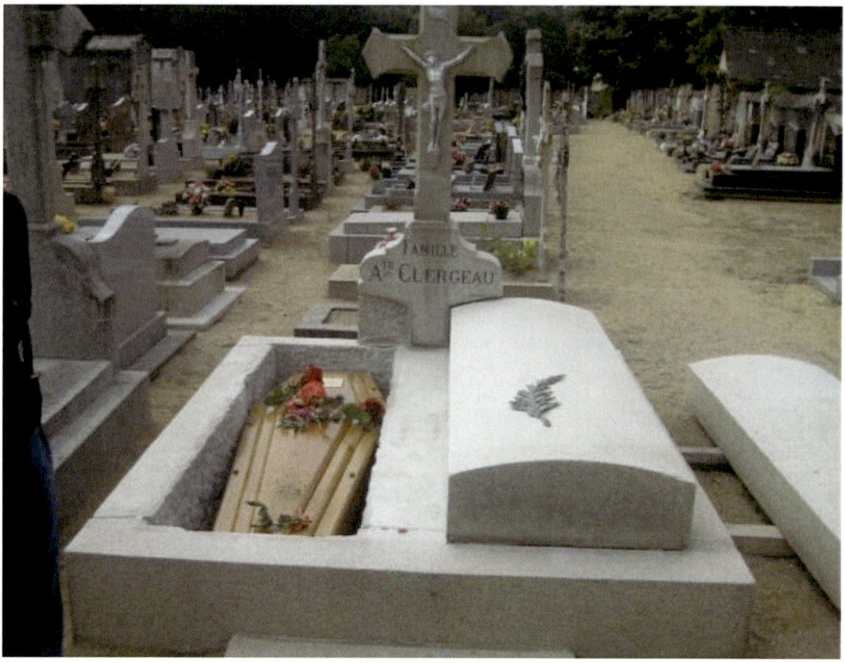

Tessier being laid to rest in the family plot of the graveyard of the church just across the street from the family home, *Bonne Hygié*. His coffin actually arrived the day before and was too long to fit in the tomb.

The graveyard workers said that it was against French law to cut anything in a graveyard, so he was parked overnight in a nearby shed until permission could be obtained from the prefecture to cut away enough of the stone to permit placement of the casket. Tessier would have been vastly amused by the workings of French bureaucracy.

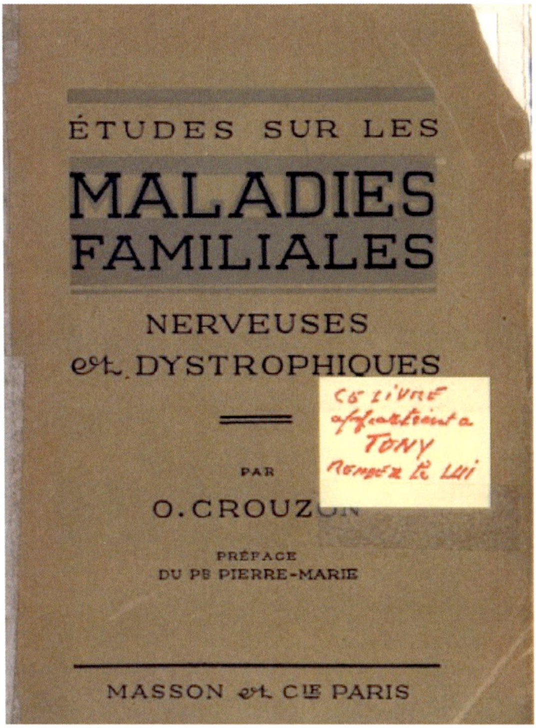

I found this book containing the original description of Crouzon's disease in the late Jim Goodrich's medical bookstore and gave it to Dr. Tessier. He refused it at first, saying I should have it and only after my insistence did he accept it. After his death, Mireille asked me to go through his library and I found the book with a Post-It saying, "This book belongs to Tony. Give it back to him."

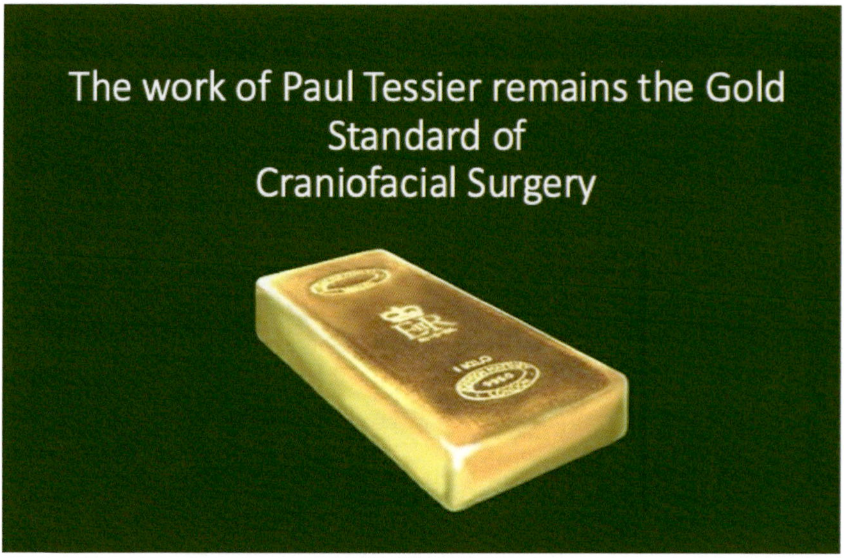

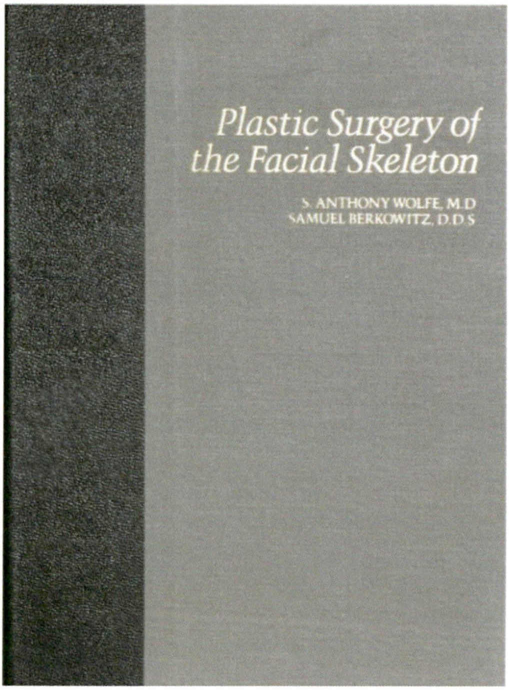

So many patients with craniofacial malformations have occlusal malformations that I asked our main orthodontist, Sam Berkowitz, to coauthor my 1989 book.

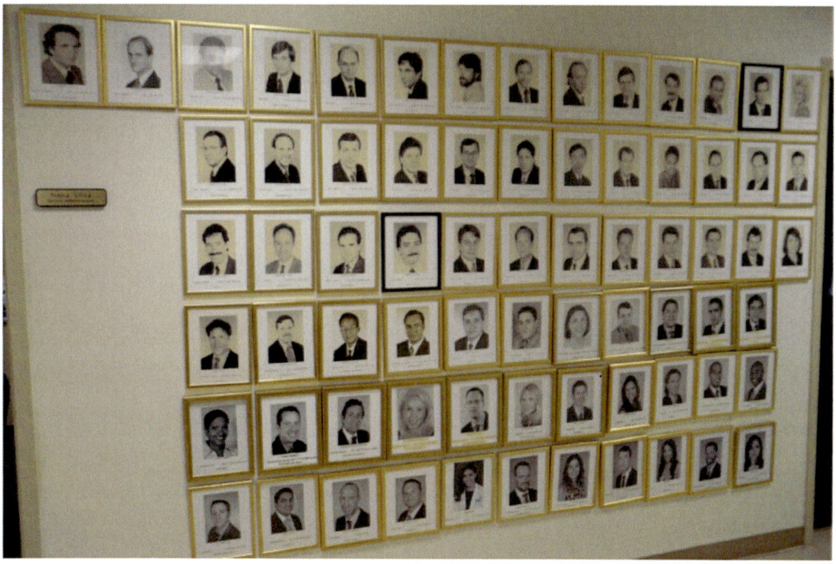

The 75 fellows we have trained since 1983 at The University of Miami and Miami (now Nicklaus) Children's Hospital. I hope I have been able to pass on to them some of what I learned from Dr. Tessier.

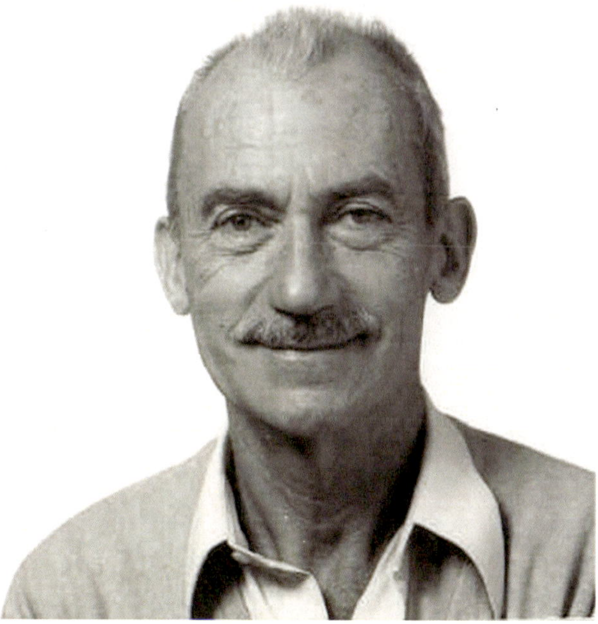

My favorite picture of Dr. Tessier, taken by Jean Claude de Wolf, life partner of Andreé Colleson, Tessier's anesthesiologist. It shows warmth, compassion, strength, and understanding, and much more.

Epilogue

We have looked at the contributions of two remarkable surgeons who have, through their innovations and contributions, changed the specialty of plastic surgery. They were both audacious and disruptive, creative and innovative, ignored and initially not accepted by their own countrymen.

Millard was not accepted into the Cleft Team at the University of Miami, and was denied the Presidency of ASPRS by a clique of Southern California aesthetic surgeons who changed the time of the business meeting without notifying the entire membership. Certainly there was an element of jealousy, because Millard's results were so good, and they were always presented with a degree of showmanship..

Tessier faced his own attempts to hold him back, from Ginestet at Foch to a shamefully delayed awarding of the Legion d'Honneur in 2005. He had already been nominated a decade earlier for the Nobel Prize by Joe Murray. Witness also the chicanery involved to prevent him from caring for Jacqueline Auriole.

There were thus similarities between the two. There were differences as well. One might say that Millard was the master of soft tissue and Tessier of hard tissue, but one must recall Tessier's superb results with eyelid burns, eyelid reconstruction and socket reconstruction where he was clearly the world leader.

Millard leaves a legacy of attention to detail and insistence that a reconstructive result be aesthetic. He was a leading aesthetic surgeon, as well as a master of reconstructive surgery. He shouldered considerable criticism from the general surgery community for his pioneering breast reconstructions.

Millard extended the existing field of plastic surgery, Tessier on the other hand created an entirely new specialty—craniofacial surgery, where he single handedly developed all of the procedures and the specialized instrumentation to make them possible.

Both men received the highest honors given by plastic surgery - Honorary Fellowship of the Royal College of Surgeons and every other organization in plastic surgery.

I was with Dr. Tessier when a reporter came by to ask for his opinion on the partial face transplant that had just been performed by the team at Amiens headed by Bernard DeVauchelle. He replied that he could not give an opinion since he had never been involved in one. However, facial transplantation with large composite segments would never have been possible without craniofacial surgery and will not become a commonplace procedure until further advances are made to safely prevent rejection. There will still be a place for classical plastic surgery as developed by Gillies, Millard, and Tessier.

Thanks to Dr. Tessier, all of the children who were put on display at the Fernald School for the Harvard Medical Students in 1964 could now receive treatment, and a normal face in all cases without face transplantation.

www.ingramcontent.com/pod-product-compliance
Lightning Source LLC
LaVergne TN
LVRC080205220926
848482LV00007B/340

* 9 7 9 8 8 8 7 2 9 4 3 0 8 *